LIQUID CONSPIRACY 2

The CIA, MI6 and Big Pharma's War on Psychedelics

Xaviant Haze

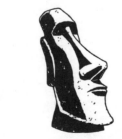

Adventures Unlimited Press

Also by Xaviant Haze

•Elvis Lives!
•Ancient Aliens in the Bible
•Robot Zombies (with Estrella Equino)
•The Suppressed History of American Banking
•Aliens in Ancient Egypt
•The Suppressed History of Ancient America

http://xavianthaze.blogspot.com

LIQUID CONSPIRACY 2

The CIA, MI6 and Big Pharma's War on Psychedelics

Xaviant Haze

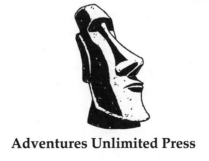

Adventures Unlimited Press

Liquid Conspiracy 2

by Xaviant Haze

Copyright © 2017

All Rights Reserved

ISBN 978-1-939149-86-2

Published by:
Adventures Unlimited Press
One Adventure Place
Kempton, Illinois 60946 USA
auphq@frontiernet.net

www.AdventuresUnlimitedPress.com

LIQUID CONSPIRACY 2

The CIA, MI6 and Big Pharma's War on Psychedelics

Xaviant Haze

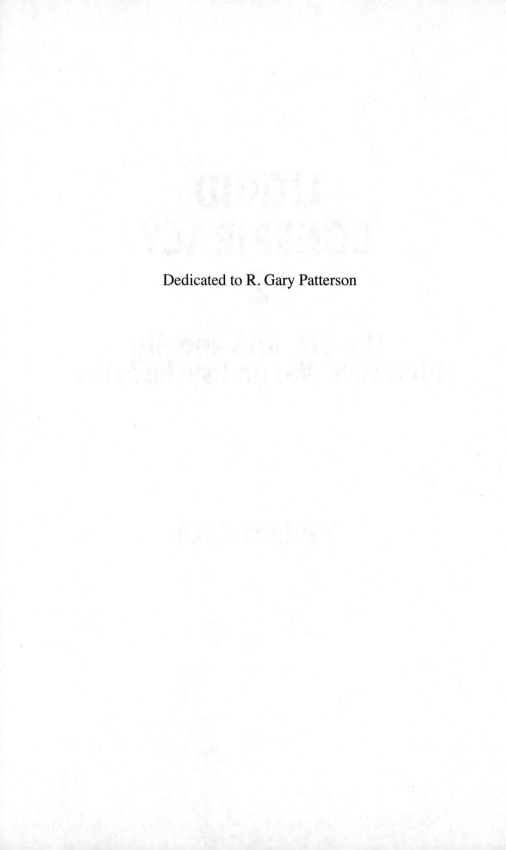

Dedicated to R. Gary Patterson

Table of Contents

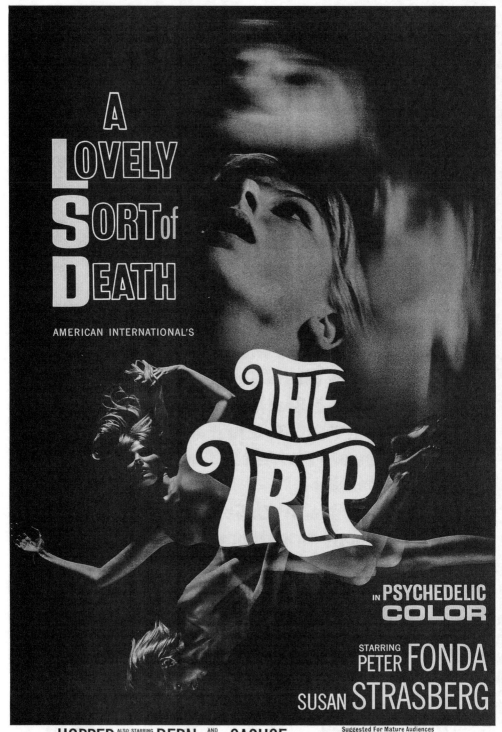

The Trip, 1967 (American International Pictures)

Introduction

Always that same LSD story, you've all seen it. 'Young man on acid, thought he could fly, jumped out of a building. What a tragedy.' What a dick! Fuck him, he's an idiot. If he thought he could fly, why didn't he take off on the ground first? Check it out. You don't see ducks lined up to catch elevators to fly south—they fly from the ground, ya moron, quit ruining it for everybody. He's a moron, he's dead—good, we lost a moron, fuckin' celebrate. Wow, I just felt the world get lighter. We lost a moron! I don't mean to sound cold, or cruel, or vicious, but I am, so that's the way it comes out. Professional help is being sought. How about a positive LSD story? Wouldn't that be news-worthy, just the once? To base your decision on information rather than scare tactics and superstition and lies? I think it would be news-worthy. 'Today, a young man on acid realized that all matter is merely energy condensed to a slow vibration. That we are all one consciousness experiencing itself subjectively. There is no such thing as death, life is only a dream and we're the imagination of ourselves' ... 'Here's Tom with the weather.'
—Bill Hicks

In the summer of 1997, the Peruvian Candyman burst through the door of my flat on 85th & Harding Ave—on the then grimy, smoked out lands of North Beach. He had a gift for my hippie soul, a tab of acid scored from some frat boys at the University of Miami. He assured me that I would be tripping balls. I only had to think it about for a split second before I popped the hit of acid on my tongue and continued to go about the business of whatever it was I was doing. I had trusted the Candyman, he was Peruvian and upon meeting him for the first time he took me to his condo in Surfside overlooking the ocean, where we talked music, ate a few magic mushrooms and watched Zeppelin's *The Song Remains the Same*

9

while figuring out the plans for the night. It wasn't any surprise that eventually he dumped a bunch of coke on the living room table, chopped up some lines and proudly declared, "Only Peruvians have glass coffee tables..." as he began to snort away.

Months later I would be sampling some high-grade college LSD in the mystical neon night of South Beach. It was my first tripping experience outside of Washington state and the first since my last trip sometime in high school. Although I had tripped a few times since my first Doors inspired outing at 16, this would be my very first acid trip that hit me on a metaphysical level. Enhanced no doubt by the wavy neon lights and art deco architecture, I found that South Beach was a perfect setting for a magically good acid trip. Scenery and mood are very important elements when determining a good or a bad trip, and apparently that night in South Beach was meant to be a transforming one. An unveiling and shedding of skin, so to speak, as I wrote poetry to the sunset on the beach like a pirate Jim Morrison.

It was a long trip and eventually I watched the sunrise float over the ocean, subatomically knowing that I would never be the same. Twenty years later, after having published over a dozen books that run the gauntlet of conspiracy lore, I get approached to write a sequel to an out of print book about psychedelic conspiracies. Apparently, the publisher wanted more material exposing the links between the CIA and psychedelic drugs like LSD, so they figured that I, being crazy enough to research and write about anything, could get the job done.

So here we are, penning another conspiracy themed tale full of the usual CIA shenanigans and deep state skullduggery. Only this time there's a light at the end of the tunnel. You see, for decades they've been pushing their propaganda about psychedelics and how dangerous and harmful they are. You might jump out of a window and slice up your mother thinking that you're peeling potatoes or some shit. Unfortunately, this might have happened a few times throughout the long history of psychedelics but let's just chalk those up to mental illness issues okay? The real truth is that scientists and therapists are discovering the profound ways psychedelic drugs can be used for treatments of all sorts of mental and health problems like PTSD and alcoholism. And with a serious fight against big pharma in the coming years, the reality of a psychedelic medical renaissance is a true possibility.

As for the *trip* you're about to embark on by reading this book, your views on the counterculture and the music of the 60s will be forever altered once you learn about the shady origins of the hippie movement that began in the CIA-monitored hills of Laurel Canyon. As for the true merchants of psychedelics it won't shock anyone to find their origins in some secret government laboratory, despite Hofmann's infamous bike ride. The British version of the CIA, known as the MI6 also had a hand in experimenting with psychedelics on their people during the flower power era. From troops to civilians, nobody was safe from the military's mad scientists behind the curtains; they even sprayed LSD on a sleepy little French town to see if it could be used as a mind control weapon of war.

The histories of psychedelics and top secret government agencies go hand in hand from the very beginning. No serious study of this shady partnership would be possible without the groundbreaking book *Acid Dreams*. Published in 1985, and written by activist authors and researchers Martin A. Lee and Bruce Shlain, the book exposed the psychedelic revolution that was spawned by LSD had its direct roots in practices and policies implanted by the CIA. LSD, the powerful force that connected so many to the organic mysteries of a universal live conscious universe turns out to have had its roots in secret CIA projects looking for truth serums, producing frightening scenarios like CIA spooks using LSD and electroshock treatments on torture victims and prisoners. They even used it on themselves, unsuspecting troops and even tried to control the experiment when acid hit the streets,—"turning on" hundreds of thousands of people in the heyday of the sixties. After plowing through thousands of pages of declassified intelligence documents and watching countless hours of congressional and

senate hearings on the connections between secret government agencies and the history of psychedelics like LSD, it becomes clear that the most paranoid and outlandish theories of the sixties pale in comparison with the actual truth.

If American citizens were paranoid in the 60s and 70s and worried about "the man," one could imagine how shocked they'd be to learn that "the man" knows everything about you now thanks to Google searches, in a world far beyond George Orwell's wildest dreams. But the rise of psychedelics arrived in a different era of American history, complete with fantastic comic book characters like Captain Al Hubbard, Aldous Huxley, Timothy Leary and others who lent a vivacious collective of LSD-inspired consciousness, that despite being illegal and opposed by the CIA, army intelligence and the deep state managed to change the face of America forever. The metaphysical windows that LSD and other psychedelics opened, lay at the heart of why the global elite continues its efforts to keep them shut. It's a war on spirituality. Much like the reason they continue to keep marijuana illegal—because it breaks the mind control, not because it's dangerous. It's the same thing for psychedelics and once they discovered how useful the drugs could be in exposing the dream world they've helped to enslave us in, they quickly moved to demonize and outlaw them. But it's too late now, as a new living cosmos pouring through the filters of the matrix have forever been exposed.

The wormhole opening was real and the psychological, sociological, scientific and political effects of LSD on American culture have been interwoven into pop culture since the 60s. Remember the Peter Fonda movie *The Trip*? An exploitation movie that came out in 1967 in an attempt to cash in on the popular acid craze sweeping the nation, *Easy Rider* it wasn't, and the plotless film written by Jack Nicholson was basically a reflection of his taking LSD as a coping mechanism from a divorce. Which is basically what actor Peter Fonda does as he wanders sunny California throughout the movie, made watchable thanks to the hilarious outdated Roger Corman era effects and a booming soundtrack from The Electric Flag. To his credit, Corman dropped acid before filming to make it authentic and, although campy, the film is about as pro-LSD as any ever made. It's curious to wonder what, if any, music Dr. Hofmann was listening to in 1938, when he first synthesized LSD (lysergic acid diethylamide) while investigating the chemical properties of a rye fungus for Sandoz Laboratories in Basel, Switzerland.

Searching for a circulatory stimulant compound, he concocted 24 different ergot derivatives that did nothing to the laboratory animals he was experimenting on. His 25th batch of LSD also failed to deliver the results hoped for and the vial of LSD gathered dust on his shelf, until the afternoon of April 16, 1943, more than five years later. A strange feeling led Hofmann to carry out a new study of the compound and while preparing a fresh batch of LSD he accidentally absorbed small drops on his fingers. Soon the good Doc was overwhelmed by a psychedelic onslaught. He described his first trip in his dairies as, "a remarkable but not unpleasant state of intoxication... characterized by an intense stimulation of the imagination and an altered state of awareness of the world. As I lay in a dazed condition with eyes closed there surged up from me a succession of fantastic, rapidly changing imagery of a striking reality and depth, alternating with a vivid, kaleidoscopic play of colors. This condition gradually passed off after about three hours."[1]

But Dr. Hofmann's first unexpected trip baffled him and he spent the next few days contemplating how such a small dose of LSD could have done that to him. The only way to find out more about this curious compound was to try it again. In the name of science of course, on the 19th a mere three days after his preliminary psychedelic voyage, Dr. Hofmann swallowed a millionth of an ounce of LSD thinking such a minuscule amount could in no way be more explosive than his first outing. Oh boy, was he was in for a surprise! Bicycling home with his laboratory assistant, he realized the symptoms were much stronger than before and he had a difficult time speaking coherently when trying to communicate. Hofmann recalled, "My field of vision swayed before me, and objects appeared distorted like images in curved mirrors. I had the impression of being unable to move from the spot, although my assistant told me afterwards that we had cycled at a good pace." Upon arriving home, he consulted a physician, who was ill equipped to deal with what would later be known as a "bad trip" as Hofmann didn't know if he'd soon be dead or stuck forever in the twisted corridors of the inner universe. "Occasionally I felt as if I were out of my body... I thought I had died. My 'ego' was suspended somewhere in space and I saw my body lying dead on the sofa," Hofmann recounted as his bad trip elevated into a shamanic experience full of optical effects and subsonic soundwaves humming in his ears until he fell sleep. He awoke the next morning feeling perfectly fine, convinced that his fateful discovery could be an important tool for studying the mind.

In time, Hofmann would refer to LSD as his "problem child" and was totally dumbfounded that his accidental creation had such an enormous social and cultural impact. He described the origins of LSD and his views on the drug in an interview with Michael Horowitz of *High Times*:

Horowitz: Did you have LSD in your laboratory as early as 1938?

Hofmann: Yes. At that time a number of pharmacological experiments were carried out in Sandoz 's department of pharmacology. Marked excitation was observed in some of the animals. But these effects did not seem interesting enough to my colleagues in the department. Work on LSD fell into abeyance for a number of years. As I had a strange feeling that it would be valuable to carry out more profound studies with this compound, I prepared a fresh quantity of LSD in the spring of 1943. In the course of this work, an accidental observation led me to carry out a planned self-experiment with this compound, which then resulted in the discovery of the extraordinary psychic effects of LSD.

Horowitz: What sort of drug were you trying to make when you synthesized LSD?

Hofmann: When I synthesized lysergic acid diethylamide, laboratory code name LSD-25 or simply LSD, I had planned the preparation of an analeptic compound, which means a circulatory and respiratory stimulant. Lysergic acid diethylamide is related in chemical structure to nicotinic acid diethylamide, known to be an effective analeptic.

Horowitz: Was the discovery of LSD an accident?

Hofmann: I would say that LSD was the outcome of a complex process that had its beginning in a definite concept and was followed by an appropriate synthesis that is, the synthesis of lysergic acid diethylamide—during the course of which a chance observation served to trigger a planned self-experiment, which then led to the discovery of the psychic effects of this compound.

Horowitz: Does "LSD-25" mean that the preparation of LSD with the characteristic psychoactive effects was the twenty-fifth one you made?

Hofmann: No, the number 25 behind LSD means that lysergic acid diethylamide was the twenty-fifth compound I had prepared in the series of lysergic acid amides.

Horowitz: In the published report of your first LSD experience on April 16, 1943, at 3:00 P.M. in Basel, you write of a "laboratory intoxication." Did you swallow something or breathe a vapor or did some drops of solution fall upon you?

Hofmann: No, I did not swallow anything, and I was used to working under very clean conditions, because these substances in general are toxic. You have to work very, very cleanly. Probably a trace of the solution of lysergic acid diethylamide I was crystallizing from methyl alcohol was absorbed through the skin of my fingers.

Horowitz: How big a dose did you take that first time, and what were the nature and intensity of that experience?

Hofmann: I don't know—an immeasurable trace. The first experience was a very weak one, consisting of rather small changes. It had a pleasant, fairy tale-magic theater quality. Three days later, on April 19, 1943, I made my first planned experiment with 0.25 milligrams, or 250 micrograms.

Horowitz: Did you swallow it?

Hofmann: Yes, I prepared a solution of 5 milligrams and took a fraction corresponding to 250 micrograms, or 25 millionths of a gram. I didn't expect this dose to work at all, and planned to take more and more to get the effects. There was no other substance known at the time which had any effect with so small a dose.

Horowitz: Did your colleagues know that you were making this experiment?

Hofmann: Only my assistant.

Horowitz: Were you familiar with the work done on mescaline by Klüver, Beringer and Rouhier in the late 1920s before you yourself experimented with mind-altering substances?

Hofmann: No—I became interested in their work only

after the discovery of LSD. They are pioneers in the field of psychoactive plants. Mescaline, studied for the first time by Lewin in 1888, was the first hallucinogen available as a chemically pure compound; LSD was the second. Karl Beringer's investigations were published in the classic monograph Der Meskalinrausch in 1928, but in the years following, interest in the hallucinogenic research faded. Not until my discovery of LSD, which is about 5,000 to 10,000 times more active than mescaline, did this line of research receive a new impetus.

Horowitz: Did government agents aware of LSD approach you during World War II?

Hofmann: Before Werner Stoll's psychiatric report appeared in 1947, there was no general knowledge of LSD. In military circles in the 1950s, however, there was open discussion of LSD as an "incapacitating drug" and thus "a weapon without death." At that time the U.S. Army sent a representative to Sandoz to speak to me about the procedure for producing large quantities of LSD.[2]

Hofmann later believed that perhaps LSD was a divine antidote to the nuclear curse the scientists at the Manhattan Project put on humanity, and that it would blaze a trail to a global psychedelic awakening that could avert future wars and destruction. LSD as a chemical messiah isn't so far-fetched as it provides a breaking of the mental straitjacket that society imposes on everyone. As we move towards a technologically driven worldwide police state, the more people without access to psychedelics to raise their consciousness and to see through the matrix, the stronger the censorship-tipped iron fist of mind control becomes. But you don't need LSD to break through the matrix, a good Wi-Fi connection and access to Youtube will get the layers of reality to begin to peel away.

You can watch almost anything you can think of including Senate hearings from the 80s where Ted Kennedy, then chairman of the Senate Subcommittee on Health and Scientific Research, attempted to bring the shady details of Operation MK-ULTRA to the public. The flagship CIA program was involved in developing chemical and biological agents for mind control purposes during the decades after World War II. Kennedy grilled a group of former CIA agents about the testing of LSD and other psychedelic drugs on unsuspecting American citizens and military personnel. Declassified documents later explained why the program was kept secret:

> The knowledge that the Agency is engaging in unethical and illicit activities would have serious repercussions in political and diplomatic circles and would be detrimental to the accomplishment of its mission.[3]

Kennedy wasn't looked upon favorably by the CIA, who viewed him as a public nuisance after basically whacking his older brothers Bobby and Jack. Ted Kennedy's war with the CIA wasn't as deadly (for him) and despite outing a few details concerning their past mind control operations his Senate hearings turned out to be duds as the senators listened to tales of buffoonery and failed experiments that stressed the agency's ineptitude, deflecting any serious scrutiny of LSD or drug-related mishaps. Kennedy's star witness was the sorcerer himself, the CIA's chief scientist Dr. Sidney Gottlieb, the man who ran the MK-ULTRA program. Author and scholar Andrei Codrescu describes the Bronx-born spymaster and chemist Gottlieb and details the day the former head of MK-ULTRA had to kind of show up to a Senate hearing:

> Gottlieb, a slight man with short gray hair and a clubfoot, agreed to testify only after receiving a grant of immunity from criminal prosecution. His testimony before the Senate subcommittee marked the first public appearance of this shadowy figure since he left the Agency in 1973. Actually his appearance was "semi-public." Because he suffered from a heart condition, Gottlieb was allowed to speak with the senators in a small antechamber while everyone else listened to the proceedings over a public address system. The purpose of Operation MK-ULTRA and related programs, Gottlieb explained, was "to investigate whether and how it was possible to modify an individual's behavior by covert means." When asked to elaborate on what the CIA learned from this research, Gottlieb was afflicted by

17

a sudden loss of memory, as if he were under the influence of one of his own amnesia drugs. However, he did confirm earlier reports that prostitutes were used in the safehouse experiments to spike the drinks of unlucky customers while CIA operatives observed, photographed, and recorded the action. When asked to justify this activity, Gottlieb resorted to the familiar Cold War refrain that had been invoked repeatedly throughout the hearings by other witnesses. The original impetus for the CIA's drug programs, he maintained, stemmed from concern about the aggressive use of behavior-altering techniques against the US by its enemies. Gottlieb claimed there was evidence (which he never shared with the senators) that the Soviets and the Red Chinese might have been mucking about with LSD in the early 1950s. This, he explained, had grave implications for our national security. At the close of the hearings Kennedy summed up the surreptitious LSD tests by declaring, "These activities are part of history, not the current practice of the CIA." And that was as far as it went. The senators seemed eager to get the whole show over with, even though many issues were far from resolved.[4]

After the Senate hearings, a flood of documents pertaining to Operation MK-ULTRA and other CIA mind control projects were made available thanks to a Freedom of Information request by researcher John Marks. By 2017 almost three million more once classified documents were made available by the CIA. These once secret documents described CIA experiments in sensory deprivation, ESP, remote viewing, telepathic subliminal effects and other methods perfect for behavior modification and mind control, and even Zoolander-esque projects turning people into programmed assassins able to kill on command with certain trigger words. The documents repeatedly referred to exotic drugs with biological compounds that caused zombie-like symptoms, actively predicting the world in which most American live in now. A wasteland of pilled-out zombies. Beware of zombies. And when the CIA wasn't interested in exploring the limits of the mind, the agency was looking for new ways to kill you. Heart attack guns and untraceable cancer-laced boots were developed long before they thought of killing Andrew Breitbart and Bob Marley.

The agency can also add the "greatest drug dealers of all time" feather to their already feather-filled cap, as nearly every "drug" that appeared on the black market since the 1960s —marijuana, cocaine, heroin, PCP, magic mushrooms, DMT, crystal meth and loads of others—had already been tested and refined by CIA and military scientists. It's no secret that the agency dumped a bunch of crack cocaine in the inner cities of America during the 1980s. If it had been a bunch of LSD the outcome would have been much different. Those in the company who first tested LSD in the early 1950s were convinced that it would revolutionize the world of covert operations. But since it's been used as a mind control drug and a mind-expanding drug that ultimately leads to defeating the imposed mind control, something funny happened on the way to the forum. This LSD-25 as it's technically termed has a covert history, rooted in CIA and military experiments with hallucinogens that started in the early 1950s with Project BLUEBIRD. Somehow the agency obtained the LSD, maybe even from Hofmann himself who might have worked in secret for the CIA.

A decade after the CIA acquired it, LSD exploded into pop culture prominence culminating in a psychedelic movement that changed the cultural landscape. Flash forward from the 1960s to the 21st century where we live in a world still engulfed by the lies, propaganda and agendas driven by the CIA with the hopes of mind controlling the sheep into submission. Psychedelic "drugs" are still illegal and thought crimes that go against the grain of the mainstream might put you in jail. Drops of acid, tokes of weed and all other matrix breaking psychedelics will also put you in jail if you get caught with them in almost 90% of the world. In some countries like Saudi Arabia they might even chop your head off! Let that sink in. What are the global elites that rule humanity so afraid of? *Liquid Conspiracy 2* will attempt to bring the complete true story of the CIA, the MI6 and Big Pharma's war on psychedelics full circle, and in the process help expose a new generation to the psychedelic renaissance that never ended.

DRAFT- ▓▓▓▓ *A*
9 June 1953

MEMORANDUM FOR THE RECORD

SUBJECT: Project MKULTRA, Subproject 8

    1. Subproject 8 is being set up as a means to continue the
present work in the general field of L.S.D. at ▓▓▓▓▓▓▓▓▓▓ *B*
▓▓▓▓ until 11 September 1954.

    2. This project will include a continuation of a study of the
biochemical, neurophysiological, sociological, and clinical psychiatric
aspects of L.S.D., and also a study of L.S.D. antagonists and drugs
related to L.S.D., such as L.A.E. A detailed proposal is attached.
The principle investigators will continue to be ▓▓▓▓▓▓▓▓▓▓ *a*
C ▓▓▓▓▓▓▓▓▓▓▓▓▓▓▓▓▓▓ all of ▓▓▓▓▓▓▓▓▓▓▓▓ *B*
-B

    3. The estimated budget of the project at ▓▓▓▓▓▓▓▓ *B*
▓▓▓ is $39,500.00. The ▓▓▓▓▓▓▓▓▓▓▓▓▓▓ will serve as a *B*
cut-out and cover for this project and will furnish the above funds
to the ▓▓▓▓▓▓▓▓▓▓▓▓▓▓▓ as a philanthropic grant for *B*
medical research   A service charge of $790 00 (2% of the estimated

Memorandum for Project MKULTRA on LSD

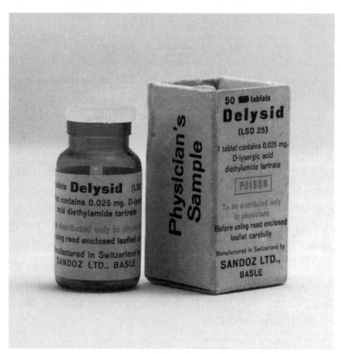

Vintage Sandoz LSD bottle with box (*Reddit*)

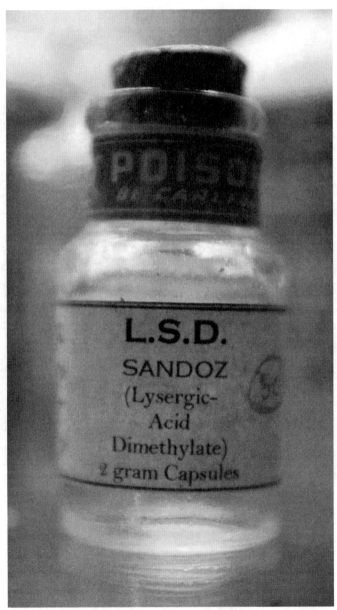

Vintage Sandoz LSD bottle (*Pinterest*)

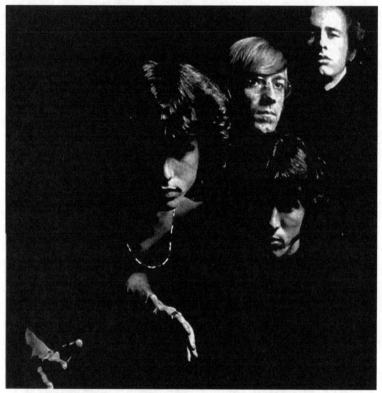

The Doors debut album photo session (*Joel Brodsky*)

Chapter One

The Pioneers of Psychedelia

Objects and their functions no longer had any significance. All I perceived was perception itself, the hell of forms and figures devoid of human emotion and detached from the reality of my unreal environment. I was an instrument in a virtual world that constantly renewed its own meaningless image in a living world that was itself perceived outside of nature. And since the appearance of things was no longer definitive but limitless, this paradisiacal awareness freed me from the reality external to myself. The fire and the rose, as it were, became one.
—Federico Fellini

My first psychedelic trip was precipitated by the usual boredom of high school, when I left for lunch with a bunch of rockers and didn't return to class. Instead we opted to catch a ride across town to a dilapidated old Victorian home rotting away somewhere in South Tacoma. Upon entering the house, we were greeted by a throng of cats and the barking of what sounded like a huge dog nestled somewhere in the back. We heard a calling for us from upstairs and I followed the line of rockers up a narrow staircase that led to the second floor. The electric sounds of a live guitar summoned us all to a large bedroom, where we gathered on bean bags or the floor, watching our host strum away on his Fender, which was riddled with stickers of punk bands and marijuana leaves.

Our dealer was your typical 80s metalhead that had the looks, yet fame and glory eluded him. And even though grunge rock and acts like Nirvana were now taking over, dude clung to his delusions of metal grandiosity of a bygone era, one he was sure would reappear—it never did. He put his guitar down just long enough to sell us a bag of sticky Washington green and then, after shoving the money in his pocket, grabbed his guitar and went into a rendition of—what else—"Money" from Pink Floyd. This of course sparked the famous conversation that starts with, "Did you know that if you watch *The Wizard of Oz* while listening to *The Dark Side of the Moon* they totally sync up with each and it blows your mind? The guy who engineered the album was trippin' on acid and watching Oz while mixing and mastering. You should totally eat some acid and see if it's true."

I had heard this rumor before and while my other rocker amigos didn't seem to show much interest, I was intrigued to learn more and although I had no idea who this dude was, I figured anyone looking this *cool* probably knows what he's talking about. "Have you done it?" I asked him as he took a long drag off the joint that was currently floating around. "Of course man, a few times, also watched *The Wall*… shit dude the entire Pink Floyd library is built around acid. Perfect for trippin' balls. Also check out The Doors…" my brain was furiously making notes inside my head as he listed a bunch of other prime suspects to get into while trippin' and when he finally stopped talking long enough I butted in and asked, "Do you have any acid?" to which he smiled and said, "A ticket to ride is $10 buckaroos my man." I paid and watched him rummage around some boxes on his shelf, from which he came back with a sheet of acid in the resemblance of the face of Jesus. He broke off a piece of Jesus' eye and told me to put it on my tongue. I did. We continued to smoke some more weed and before I knew it we were all squished inside the car, a green Pinto, cruising towards school, where everyone got out except me and the driver. He had some acid too, and suggested we go to his house where we could test this Pink Floyd theory. I wasn't feeling anything at that point and figured the whole thing to be buillshit. When we arrived at his house, we made a beeline for the basement where the stereo and television were set up near a series of old couches.

Soon we were watching *The Wizard of Oz* while listening to *The Dark Side of the Moon*, convinced that the syncing of the two wasn't some coincidence. By the time we watched *The Wall* both of us were totally trippin' to the point that we started to panic just a bit. I left for dinner and despite the long walk was able to make it home in time not to get rained on. That walk resembled a Stephen

King painting in a way only those from the Pacific Northwest might understand: an endless sky of grey, host to misshapen clouds that torment you with their refusal to rain. And although I escaped getting wet, I couldn't escape getting the key into the keyhole— *Why was the door locked? Was it that late?* After what seemed like forever scratching the key around the keyhole my annoyed aunt let me inside. I dashed upstairs and hid in my bedroom; laying on the bed and staring up at the ceiling I had my first hallucination.

A series of silverware, forks and spoons and such, all floating down in a straight line. Was this my gut telling my subconscious mind that it was time to eat? I was indeed hungry but unaware of how to approach the kitchen and the act of eating while on acid. After wrestling around on the bed for a few while trying to shake off the hallucinations I was finally able to muster up enough courage for a run to the kitchen. I avoided everyone and somehow managed to make a peanut butter and jelly sandwich without destroying the kitchen or myself. I ate it upstairs in my room and began phase two of my trip. I put on The Doors—basically my teenage life changed forever afterwards as I became obsessed with Jim Morrison. And you would too if he had performed in a black robe on your bedroom wall in a private performance only available once during your first acid trip. So, my first trip ended with a private, robe-clad performance from the lizard king himself, not bad.

Jim Morrison and his band the Doors helped usher in the era of psychedelia but the true pioneers of LSD were entrepreneurial misfits and dissatisfied scientists beholden to intelligence agencies. The real "Captain Trips" wasn't Jerry Garcia or the name of the plague that killed almost everybody in Stephen King's *The Stand*, it was Al Hubbard, a former OSS Captain who rode around in a Rolls-Royce and made millions selling uranium. A true insider, he hung with the who's who of the illuminati, visited Bohemian Grove and was considered the Johnny Appleseed of LSD. His friends called him "Cappy" and he loved drinking Bahamian rum, fishing and turning people on to LSD. He's regarded as the first person to promote LSD as a positive transcendental drug and made it his life's mission to hip the public to its benefits, much to the dismay of his fellow illuminati brethren.

Captain Trips Hubbard believed that most people were walking in their sleep and needed a good dose of LSD to wake up and see themselves for what they are. Words of advice from a former spy who laundered several million dollars through the American consulate in Vancouver to finance covert operations in Europe during the rise of World War II. The Captain was turned on to LSD by the English chemist Dr. Ronald Sandison in 1951, where during his trip he claimed to have witnessed the perversion of his own conception. Hubbard, then almost fifty, sought out British psychiatrist Dr. Humphry Osmond, who was working with LSD and mescaline at Weyburn Hospital in Saskatchewan, Canada. The CIA was also snooping around the hospital, spending the next decade closely monitoring Osmond's psychedelic progress. Before Hubbard came, Osmond, a young psychiatrist, was struggling to find a cure for alcoholism. He hadn't viewed LSD as a possible treatment until the Captain showed him how to harness its transcendent potential. Almost a thousand alcoholics were given LSD treatment with more than half responding favorably to the cure. Osmond couldn't believe it, and wondered if LSD could be the most important drug in psychiatric history. He also wondered if it could save the world. With the help of Captain Trips the well-connected duo set up a series of private acid trips with some of the most influential politicians of the time including prime ministers, heads of state, members of Congress and members of the British parliament. Soon, Hubbard and Osmond became psychedelic shrinks who plied business and political leaders with copious amounts of acid and asked them questions while strobe lights paraded off the walls.

The good Captain zigzagged across America with over six thousand bottles of LSD during the 1950s in an attempt to turn people on from all walks of life. He even had his own plane that he traveled around the world with buying up and stashing LSD, sometimes flying the plane himself as he greeted those in need of the psychedelic wonder drug. In Los Angeles, the Captain was the toast of the town at social gatherings in the mid-1950s as his LSD-inspired congregations of scientists, philosophers and intellectuals provided an eclectic mix of personalities. Hubbard was an intelligence agent, and one wonders what he was really up to—was it more than just a love affair with LSD?

Hubbard never officially joined the rebranded agency after

his stint with the OSS ended, and he bitterly complained that the company owed him millions in back pay. He also didn't like what the CIA was doing with his beloved LSD, as they dismissed his offerings of help and used the drug with sinister intentions. And although he was 'one of the boys' so to speak, the Captain knew that even he was expendable if the deep state willed it. To stay within their good graces, he engaged in undercover work for the Food and Drug Administration and maintained employment at Teledyne, a CIA asset and major defense contractor. The rebel Captain was an unlikely enigma, a redneck mystic that rose to the highest levels of the pyramid despite maintaining an outsider's stance. Some claim that Hubbard knew more about LSD than anyone else in the world and maybe he did; one things for certain—he wasn't shy about sharing.

Aldous Huxley benefited from the Captain's graciousness, taking his first LSD trip upon meeting Hubbard for a session in 1953 in the Hollywood Hills. With the Captain guiding him, Huxley took his first tiny dose of LSD, an experience about which he proclaimed, "What came through the closed door was the realization—not the knowledge, for this wasn't verbal or abstract—but the direct, total awareness, from the inside, so to say, of Love as the primary and fundamental cosmic fact."[1] Huxley, the prophetic British writer, and his redneckian LSD mentor made the most hilarious and improbable duo. Yet despite their different styles both shared an appreciation of the therapeutic aspects of hallucinogenic drugs. Huxley was obsessed with the ideas of a drug-induced culture owned by mind control. In 1931 Huxley wrote *Brave New World*, then a futuristic vision of a totalitarian society chemically coerced into loving its own servitude. Today, his vision is a frightening reality as statues are being torn down in the name of political correctness by drug-induced zombies. Beware of zombies.

While Huxley questioned the aspects of a society stripped of its freedoms under pharmacological attacks, he also recognized that hallucinogens could effect positive changes in consciousness. He wrote about his personal psychedelic experiences in *The Doors of Perception*, where he claimed that the screening mechanisms of the matrix can be suspended with the help of mescaline and LSD. Huxley believed that when administered in the right environment,

27

psychedelics can lead to mystical and religious experiences, and envisioned a world that operated on a higher level because of the drugs. He even requested a shot of LSD on his deathbed, and went to the afterlife tripping. Huxley also fought against the CIA's goals for the drug which were to impose an altered state on its victims to control them, instead of using it as mind expanding tool for loving humanity and nature. Although Huxley was aware of the dangers of behavior modification techniques via psychedelic means he was good friends with some of the greatest mind control scientists, ever like Dr. J. West, an MK-ULTRA scientist that conducted LSD studies for the CIA, and J. B. Rhine, director of ESP studies for the CIA. While writing *Heaven and Hell* in 1955, Huxley began to wonder if the scientific approach was utterly hopeless as the view of the drug in the academic circles wasn't favorable and the ill-willed agendas of the deep state threatened the possibility of a psychedelic utopia.

But the pioneers of psychedelia stretch back to the ancient shamans of Native America who sipped and tripped on their mystical peyote potions while the magic mushrooms of the ancient Vedic cultures were gobbled up in northern India. The ancient Greeks loved ergot (LSD's cousin) thousands of years ago, where it was called kykeon and used in sacred mystery rites. The party ended when the Christians came to power in the 4th century and banned any future parties inspired by the elysian ergot fields of psychedelic joys:

> When Christianity was adopted as the official creed of the Roman Empire in the fourth century, all other religions, including the Mysteries, were banished. Christian propagandists called for the destruction of the pagan drug cults that had spread throughout Europe after the Roman conquest. Like its shamanistic forebears, paganism was rooted in rapture rather than faith or doctrine; its mode of expression was myth and ritual, and those who carried on the forbidden traditions possessed a vast storehouse of knowledge about herbs and special medicaments. The witches of the Middle Ages concocted brews with various hallucinogenic compounds—belladonna, thorn apple,

henbane and bufotenine (derived from the sweat gland of the toad Bufo marinus) —and when the moon was full they flew off on their imaginary broomsticks to commune with spirits.[2]

Now outlawed, these rites of the Eleusinian Mysteries, went underground where they remained the oldest psychedelic pagan religion in the West. This secret ceremony that culminated in a mass tripping inspired pilgrims from all over the world to take part in its ritual centered on the drinking of the sacred ergot-laced kykeon brew:

> After drinking the spiritual potion, the initiates would listen to ceremonial music and ponder the texts of Demeter, goddess of grain (symbolizing renewal, spring, fecundity, and possibly the ergot fungus, which grows on barley, from which the kykeon was made). At the climax of the initiation a beam of sunlight would flood the chamber. This vision was said to be the culminating experience of a lifetime, man's redemption from death. As the poet Pindar wrote, "Happy is he who, having seen these rites, goes below the hollow earth; for he knows the end of life and its god-sent beginning." Plato, Aristotle and Sophocles were among those who participated in this secret ritual. While the passing of time and the destruction of documentary evidence by the church has concealed the full scope of the ritual use of hallucinogens in Europe, scattered references suggest that a widespread psychedelic underground existed during the Middle Ages.[3]

By the time European "witchcraft" was stamped out by the Holy Inquisition, the conquistadors were eradicating peyote, kava, marijuana and coca leaves used by the indigenous natives in the Americas as part of an imperialist effort to remove all access to the psychedelic experience. This worked until the poets and artists discovered the joys of laudanum, a tincture of opium that dominated high society London of the late eighteenth century. Those dastardly drugs had once again been infused into culture as the literary likes of Edgar Allan Poe and Victor Hugo, who both viewed society as a torturous bummer, often used drugs to escape society while writing groundbreaking literary works under the influence.

As the 50s ended, the CIA-fronted Josiah Macy, Jr. Foundation sponsored the first international conference on LSD therapy. Led by Dr. Paul Hoch, the conference was a gathering of the most important LSD researchers and scientists of the time. It was also infested with company men like Dr. Harold Abramson, a veteran of the MK-ULTRA program, and several other scientists like Hoch who worked with the CIA and other defense contractors beholden to the military industrial complex. Dr. Hoch wasn't onboard as far as to say that LSD could be helpful as a therapeutic tool and essentially dubbed all psychedelic drugs as anxiety-producing menaces unfit for human consumption. However, almost all his peers were unanimous in believing that LSD could be very beneficial as most patients found the drug to be amazing enough to want to try again. Hoch never tried LSD or mescaline, instead he opted to experiment with it on mental patients who were given the drugs while being tortured with electroshock therapy. Hoch even ordered lobotomies and did post-lobotomy testing with psychedelics on the poor patients. Dr. Hoch was basically just another monster working for the CIA who wielded a large wand of authority as his views on hallucinogenic drugs would become the blueprint talking points for the media to now parrot—that psychedelics were extremely dangerous and can you drive you batshit insane. Both the mainstream media and the medical establishment began to promote this "LSD is bad mm'kay" mantra—much like they did with the fear mongering reefer madness campaigns of 30s and 40s, much to the delight of the CIA. By promoting LSD in a damaging negative light, LSD would forever be seen as illegal and dangerous by the FDA, DEA and the police state patrols of the future. And while getting busted for a hit of acid may seem like something that only happened to hippies in the 60s, the truth is that if you happen to be caught today with the psychedelic wonder you'd end up in prison with a felony record much the same. But how did LSD go from a lab in Switzerland to the sunny coasts of California anyway? The same way you and I might go down to Walgreens and refill our prescriptions—with $$$.

Basically, the CIA sent a few guys to Sandoz Laboratories in

Basel with a suitcase of money where they proceeded to buy up the world's supply of LSD. Replacing the money with bottles of the drug in their suitcases, the agents easily brought the LSD back to America safe and secure and without the hassle of the TSA or anyone else to bother them. From that supply the company began their top secret mind control program now known as MK-ULTRA in which they had not only LSD to play with but a cornucopia of all sorts of other so-called drugs. With the rise of a new counterculture on its way, the CIA was at ground zero of planting the seeds of a new drug war that saw the prohibition of psychedelics at any cost, while at the same being responsible for facilitating and expanding the trade and use of the very drugs it's supposedly trying to stamp out. As of 2017, it's no longer a secret that the CIA and the DEA are essentially the biggest drug dealers in the world, in a scam that benefits only themselves, cartels, criminals and the prison industrial complex which gets prisoners for slave labor at 50 cents an hour. It's this massive prison labor force that has kept the minimum wage pay at the lowest levels in order to compete with the high output, low overhead of the prison slave labor factories.[4] But back in the early 50s the company was worried that those pesky Russians had already started using LSD as a truth serum on potential spies and were in a rush to get in on the action.

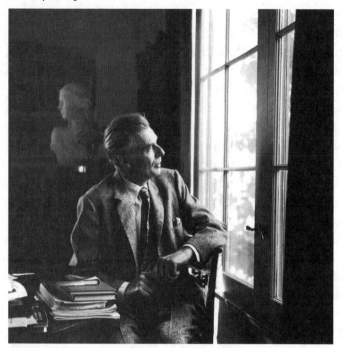

Aldous Huxley (*Pinterest*)

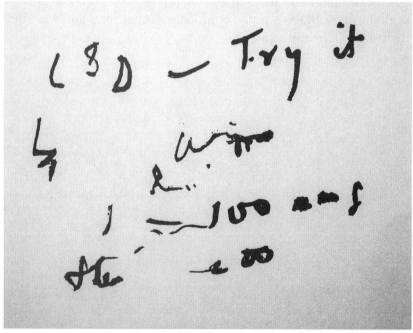

Aldous Huxley's final note to his wife Laura: "LSD, 100 mcg, intramuscular – Try it."

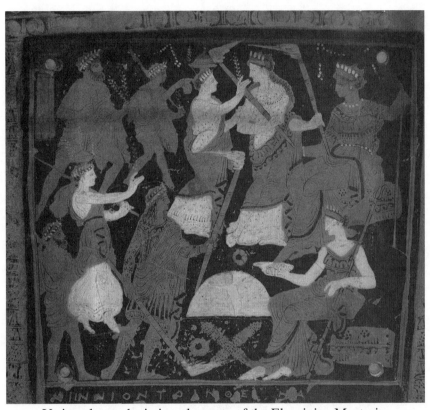

Votive plaque depicting elements of the Eleusinian Mysteries
(*Carole Raddato*)

Chapter Two

Operations BLUEBIRD and ARTICHOKE

In the end the Controllers realized that force was no good.
The slower but infinitely surer methods ...neo-Pavlovian
conditioning and hypnopaedia ...Accompanied by a
campaign against the Past; by the closing of museums, the
blowing up of historical monuments... by the suppression
of all books published before A.F. 150.
– Aldous Huxley, *Brave New World*

The bummer of a bad trip can't truly be explained to the uninitiated, it must be experienced by the conduit inhabiting the trip and successfully illustrated coherently to a later audience. My first bad trip occurred shortly after my first good trip somewhere in the memory hole of high school. It was a Friday night and we had taken the acid early in anticipation of a punk rock concert we were supposed to go to but car troubles and a neighboring gang war kept us holed up inside the house. I began to get restless and crawled into a corner of the bedroom where I tried to ignore the highlighted thumps of the helicopter blades as the ghetto bird flew over the neighborhood. The silhouettes of its wings stabbed through the crevice in the blinds and I covered my eyes and ears hoping to drown out the sound and visions. Eventually I couldn't take any more and braved my way home.

The first obstacle would be catching the bus which I somehow managed to do; the next obstacle would be getting off the bus which was harder than usual. The colored tracers of my trip, which was full speed ahead at that point, had rendered the ground I wanted to step on useless—it looked like a giant cavern 3,000 feet deep! *But I'm supposed to get off the bus.* At least according to the dumbfounded bus driver who was staring back at me with his hands up, yelling undecipherable words my direction. *But there's no ground.* I couldn't wait any longer, who knows how long I had held up the bus at the point. I closed my eyes and leaped off the bus. I can only imagine how I looked, I'm sure it was hilarious as I flailed my way towards the ground that felt like it took an eternity to land on. But at last, I was up, brushed off and could appear to walk normally as I got my wits together and began to walk home.

The red neon sign proclaiming *Jesus Lives* hung above the church and the cold cloudy winds of November signaled winter was near. I lifted up the hood of my Oakland Raiders parka, feeling its feathers warm my ears; I was almost home. The black Raiders jacket was straight from swap meet Louie with the fake starter patch sewn on the shoulder. It was badass, and a target as I soon found out when I felt the sudden tug of my hood which violently spun me around to a gun in my face. Total bummer, as I stared into the melted barrel of a snubnose 38, the glowing red eyes of its gunslinger frisking me as I wiggled my way out of the jacket. The robber took off with my coat as I watched him disappear, my trip with him—by the time I shivered my way inside the house my first bad trip only got worse as I fumbled to explain just what the hell happened. To my family I was clearly on drugs. By the time I was able to climb into bed and my put my headphones on I was well aware that the weeks ahead would somehow mimic the mojo of the bad trip I was trying to sleep off.

The first trips the military took when experimenting with drugs weren't really trips at all, they were centered around marijuana and whether it could be used as a potential truth serum for use in intelligence interrogations. It was the early 1940s and reefer madness was in full effect. So, chief of the Office of Strategic Services (OSS), the CIA's wartime predecessor—General 'Wild Bill' Donovan—gathered a few scientists and began a top secret research program revolving around drugs and secret agents. This would be the first attempt at modifying human behavior through chemical means by the OSS, a tradition that carried on well into the 21st century by the CIA. In 1942, the OSS was looking to break down the psychological defenses of enemy spies in the hope they would reveal useful, perhaps even classified information. And for some reason they thought marijuana could help them do it. The sweet leaf was chosen as the most likely candidate for a truth serum as OSS scientists created highly potent batches of concentrated cannabis in liquid form. The cannabis-infused drink had had no color, odor, or taste and was nearly impossible to detect. The agency was sure they had created the perfect truth-telling serum and thus named their new project TD as in "truth drug."

In their minds, there was no way any other friendly or rival countries like Russia could be creating the same type of cannabis-inspired drug, for the simple fact that no one else at the time had what seemed like an unlimited source of marijuana, a bountiful weed that grew almost everywhere in the American west. The agency tried various ways of administering the marijuana serum, injecting it into foods, creating cosmic brownies and edibles that unsuspecting suspects would gobble up before getting too stoned to coherently spill their guts. Most of the time the patients either fell asleep or suffered laugh attacks that stretched for hours, rendering the experiment useless. They next tried to inject the Marijuana serum into cigarettes or cigars, hoping that after smoking, the suspect would get so high that a skillful interrogator could easily get him to spill the beans. The effects of the liquid serum were described in a once classified OSS report:

> TD appears to relax all inhibitions and to deaden the areas of the brain which govern an individual's discretion and caution. It accentuates the senses and makes manifest any strong characteristics of the individual. Sexual inhibitions are lowered, and the sense of humor is accentuated to the point where any statement or situation can become extremely funny to the subject. On the other hand, a person's unpleasant characteristics may also be heightened. It may be stated that, generally speaking, the reaction will be one of great loquacity and hilarity.[1]

After testing the serum on each other and various US military personnel, the OSS finally decided that the herb wasn't a useful truth serum and any damage the drug might cause would most likely be to the refrigerator.

After the end of World War II, the Navy picked up where the OSS left off in the search for a top secret truth serum by initiating

Project CHATTER[2] in 1947. This was a pivotal year in American history, one that saw the beginning of the CIA, the crash at Roswell and the most spectacular atomic bomb tests to date. CHATTER was spearheaded at the Naval Medical Research Institute in Bethesda, Maryland by Dr. Charles Savage (a comic book villain's name if there ever was one) who conducted experiments with mescaline synthesized from peyote, a psychedelic flower that grows on the tip of a certain southwestern cactus much adored by shamans. But these mescaline-laced studies, which were also carried out on animals, failed to produce the desired results and the operation was canceled in 1953. One wonders what could possibly be learned from giving ol' fido the dog mescaline? Were they expecting him to magically be given the powers of speech?

Around the same time that CHATTER ended, the CIA was actively seeking ways to render people incoherent, truth-speaking zombies through psychological and pharmacological attacks. If they had to have their test subjects committed to mental institutions to get the job done, then so be it. Thousands of subjects were committed involuntarily to insane asylums in a CIA monitored program that spanned a decade. It's scarier than it sounds—most of the subjects were dissidents whose political views landed them in psychiatric hospitals for reprogramming. Shielded by the deep state's bureaucratic apparatus, the CIA's first mind control via drugs experiment was kicked off with Operation BLUEBIRD, a mission that skipped the Projects Review Committee and went straight to CIA director Roscoe Hillenkoetter, who authorized the untraceable funds to finance the daring experiment. BLUEBIRD was a carefully guarded secret, an operation described in one CIA document as, "not fit for public consumption" and in another as, "broad and comprehensive, involving both domestic and overseas activities, and taking into consideration the programs and objectives of other departments, principally the military services."[3] Thus, nobody was safe from BLUEBIRD's efforts to create exploitable personality alterations via chemical means. The program's name was changed to operation ARTICHOKE[4] a few years after its inception, as the search for a reliable truth-telling substance still eluded the agency. The alchemical deus ex machina was nowhere to be found and the whole idea of a truth drug seemed too good to be true:

It presupposed that there was a way to chemically bypass the mind's censor and turn the psyche inside out, unleashing a profusion of buried secrets, and that surely some approximation of "truth" would emerge amidst all the personal debris. In this respect the ClA's quest resembled a skewed version of a familiar mythological theme from which such images as the Philosopher's Stone and the Fountain of Youth derive—that through touching or ingesting something one can acquire wisdom, immortality, or eternal peace. It is more than a bit ironic that the biblical inscription on the marble wall of the main lobby at CIA headquarters in Langley, Virginia, reads, "And ye shall know the Truth and the Truth shall set you free." The freewheeling atmosphere that prevailed during the ClA's early years encouraged an "anything goes" attitude among researchers associated with the mind control program. This was before the Agency's bureaucratic arteries began to harden, and those who participated in Operation ARTICHOKE were intent on leaving no stone unturned in an effort to deliver the ultimate truth drug. A number of agents were sent on fact-finding missions to all comers of the globe to procure samples of rare herbs and botanicals.[5]

One of these trips was to the Caribbean island of Puerto Rico where the agency investigated the "stupid bush," which, according to their heavily redacted report "Exploration of Potential Plant Resources in the Caribbean Region," was characterized by the CIA as a psychogenic weed that grew on the southern coast of the island. Another psychogenic weed "information bush" also stumped the CIA scientists who left a glaring—?—next to it on the report. It's uncertain what these weeds look like and what type of information was gleaned from them as the report remains heavily blacked out. The CIA studied a pharmacopoeia of drugs in the early 50s with the hope of achieving a truth serum breakthrough. Agents even believed that cocaine could be a potential truth serum thanks to the elevated heartrates and overall talkativeness associated with the drug. But large doses of cocaine via injection proved to be too much for the subjects, usually inducing panicked states of paranoia, anxiety, and in some cases, hallucinations. Procaine, a cocaine derivative was tested on mental patients to stunning results, but none that could be helpful from an interrogation standpoint. Nevertheless, they found when injecting the drug into the frontal lobes of the brain through sets of trephine holes in the skull, that it produced spontaneous outbursts of speech from mute schizophrenics within days. The CIA's tinkering with cocaine as a truth serum was short-lived, but they would have stunning success in the wholesaling and distributing of the drug in the future. However, in the 50s the agency viewed cocaine as nothing more than nose candy, sometimes dangling off the edges of their most seasoned spies. As stated in *Acid Dreams*:

> The search for an effective interrogation technique eventually led to heroin. Not the heroin that ex-Nazi pilots under CIA contract smuggled out of the Golden Triangle in Southeast Asia on CIA proprietary airlines during the late 1940s and early 1950s nor the heroin that was pumped into America's black and brown ghettos after passing through contraband networks controlled by mobsters who moonlighted as CIA hitmen. The Agency's involvement in worldwide heroin traffic, which has been well documented in *The Politics of Heroin in Southeast Asia* by Alfred McCoy, went far beyond the scope of Operation ARTICHOKE, which was primarily concerned with eliciting information from recalcitrant subjects. However, ARTICHOKE scientists did see possible advantages in heroin as a mind control drug.[6]

CIA documents revealed that heroin was used by police and intelligence officers on a routine basis as a sort of cold turkey theory of interrogation, realizing that heroin and other habit-forming substances can be a crutch to addicts who will most likely do and say anything once the jones begins to set in. But just like all the other drugs the agency experimented with, it too was abandoned as a possible truth serum, with a list of drawbacks stretching to the moon. Eventually the only candidate left standing was the mysterious LSD-25, a substance that was a complete conundrum within scientific circles at the time. Most scientists didn't even know that it existed. Dr. Wemer Stoll, the first person to investigate the psychological properties of LSD, presented his findings to the *Swiss Archives of Neurology* in 1947. This is also discussed in *Acid Dreams*:

Stoll reported that LSD produced disturbances in perception, hallucinations, and acceleration in thinking; moreover, the drug was found to blunt the usual suspiciousness of schizophrenic patients. No unfavorable aftereffects were described. Two years later in the same journal Stoll contributed a second report entitled "A New Hallucinatory Agent, Active in Very Small Amounts." The fact that LSD caused hallucinations should not have been a total surprise to the scientific community. Sandoz first became interested in ergot, the natural source of lysergic acid, because of numerous stories passed down through the ages. The CIA inherited this ambiguous legacy when it embraced LSD as a mind control drug. An ARTICHOKE document dated October 21, 1951, indicates that acid was tested initially as part of a pilot study of the effects of various chemicals "on the conscious suppression of experimental or non-threat secrets." In addition to lysergic acid this particular survey covered a wide range of substances, including morphine, ether, Benzedrine, ethyl alcohol, and mescaline. "There is no question," noted the author of this report, "that drugs are already on hand (and new ones are being produced) that can destroy integrity and make indiscreet the most dependable individual." The report concluded by recommending that LSD be critically tested "under threat conditions beyond the scope of civilian experimentation." POWs, federal prisoners, and Security officers were mentioned as possible candidates for these field experiments. In another study designed to ascertain optimal dosage levels for interrogation sessions, a CIA psychiatrist administered LSD to "at least twelve human subjects of not too high mentality." At the outset the subjects were "told only that a new drug was being tested and promised that nothing serious or dangerous would happen to them…. During the intoxication they realized something was happening, but were never told exactly what."[7]

The agency decided that a dosage range of 100 to 150 micrograms would be safe enough to test on their subjects during mock interrogation trials without risking possible hallucinations. Initial tests were positive as one officer who was given LSD revealed a bunch of detailed military secrets. Once the LSD had worn off, the officer couldn't remember revealing the classified information and had complete amnesia regarding the trial. More favorable reports about LSD kept coming in, sparking the CIA's Office of Scientific Intelligence (OSI) to prepare a lengthy new report entitled "Potential New Agent for Unconventional Warfare" which was basically a love letter to Hofmann's problem child. It seems the agency had finally found their elusive truth serum after all as the report credits LSD "for eliciting true and accurate statements from subjects under its influence during interrogation."[8] Data from the report even suggested that LSD might help retrieve buried memories of past experiences and even provide proof of reincarnation through remote viewing. Here was a drug that could unearth painful secrets buried deep in the unconscious mind, all the while causing an amnesia blackout effect during the revealing period. To the CIA the implications of this were astounding and once the hierarchy got wind of what LSD could do the agency made sure to send some agents to the Sandoz labs to buy up all that was available. The agency went trigger happy in LSD experimentation discovering that diverse reactions often occurred when people were given LSD without forewarning. On one occasion a fellow CIA agent dosed another agent's morning coffee and sat back and watched his reactions. After about a half an hour, the dosed agent began to realize what might be happening, "He sort of knew he had it," the CIA agent recalled, "but he couldn't pull himself together. Somehow, when you know you've taken it, you start the process of maintaining your composure. But this grabbed him before he was aware, and it got away from him." The dosed agent freaked out and ran off, fleeing across Washington tripping balls while the agent responsible for his trip ran after him. "He reported afterwards," the agent continued, "that every automobile that came by was a terrible monster with fantastic eyes, out to get him personally. Each time a car passed he would huddle down against a parapet, terribly frightened. It was a real horror for him. I mean, it was hours of agony... like being in a dream that never stops—with someone chasing you."[9]

Incidents like this reaffirmed just how devastating a weapon LSD could, making the agency more enthusiastic about the drug as a series of LSD ritual hazings began. But the acid pranks got out of hand and claimed their first victim on thanksgiving, 1953, when a group of CIA and army engineers gathered for a holiday retreat at a remote hunting lodge in the Maryland countryside:

> On the second day of the meeting Dr. Gottlieb spiked the after-dinner cocktails with LSD. As the drug began to take effect, Gottlieb told everyone that they had ingested a mind-altering chemical. By that time the group had become boisterous with laughter and unable to carry on a coherent conversation. One man was not amused by the unexpected turn of events. Dr. Frank Olson, an army scientist who specialized in biological warfare research, had never taken LSD before, and he slid into a deep depression. His mood did not lighten when the conference adjourned. Normally a gregarious family man, Olson returned home quiet and withdrawn. When he went to work after the weekend, he asked his boss to fire him because he had "messed up the experiment" during the retreat. Alarmed by his erratic behavior, Olson's superiors contacted the CIA, which sent him to New York to see Dr. Harold Abramson. A respected physician, Abramson taught at Columbia University and was chief of the allergy clinic at Mount Sinai Hospital. He was also one of the CIA's principal LSD researchers and a part-time consultant to the Army Chemical Corps. While these were impressive credentials, Abramson was not a trained psychiatrist, and it was this kind of counseling his patient desperately needed. For the next few weeks Olson confided his deepest fears to Abramson. He claimed the CIA was putting something in his coffee to make him stay awake at night. He said people were plotting against him and he heard voices at odd hours commanding him to throw away his wallet—which he did, even though it contained several

uncashed checks. Dr. Abramson concluded that Olson was mired in "a psychotic state... with delusions of persecution" that had been "crystallized by the LSD experience." Arrangements were made to move him to Chestnut Lodge, a sanitarium in Rockville, Maryland, staffed by CLA-cleared psychiatrists. (Apparently other CIA personnel who suffered from psychiatric disorders were enrolled in this institution.) On his last evening in New York, Olson checked into a room at the Statler Hilton along with a CIA agent assigned to watch him. And then, in the wee hours of the morning, the troubled scientist plunged headlong through a closed window to his death ten floors below. The Olson suicide had immediate repercussions within the CIA. An elaborate cover up erased clues to the actual circumstances leading up to his death. Olson's widow was eventually given a government pension, and the full truth of what happened would not be revealed for another twenty years. Meanwhile CIA director Allen Dulles suspended the in-house testing program for a brief period while an internal investigation was conducted. In the end, Gottlieb and his team received only a mildly worded reprimand for exercising "bad judgment," but no records of the incident were kept in their personnel files which would harm their future careers. The importance of LSD eclipsed all other considerations, and the secret acid tests resumed. Gottlieb was now ready to undertake the final and most daring phase of the MKULTRA program: LSD would be given to unwitting targets in real-life situations. But who would actually do the dirty work?[10]

George Hunter White, a tough, old-fashioned narcotics officer who ran a training school for American spies during World War II, was given the job as top LSD tester for the CIA. From the get go White had plenty of room and CIA funds to run his operation, he rented an apartment in hip Greenwich Village, and transformed it into a bachelor pad with pervy two-way mirrors and surveillance equipment. White was a playboy and posing as an artist, cool and rich enough to lure people back to his pad and slip them LSD. His victims were mostly girls, who were date raped while tripping.

White's personal diary, contained the reactions to the surprise LSD experiments like, "Gloria gets horrors.... Janet sky high" while the majority of bad trips prompted him to codename the drug "stormy." In 1955, White transferred out west and set up two other bachelor pad LSD experiment houses in San Francisco. From there he initiated Operation Midnight Climax, in which prostitutes were hired to pick up men from local bars and bring them back to White's CIA-financed psychedelic bordello:

Unknowing customers were treated to drinks laced with LSD while White sat on a portable toilet behind two-way mirrors, sipping martinis and watching every stoned and kinky moment. As payment for their services the hookers received $100 a night, plus a guarantee from White that he'd intercede on their behalf should they be arrested while plying their trade. In addition to providing data about LSD, Midnight Climax enabled the CIA to learn about the sexual proclivities of those who passed through the safe-houses. White's harem of prostitutes became the focal point of an extensive CIA study of how to exploit the art of lovemaking for espionage purposes. When he wasn't operating a national security whorehouse, White would cruise the streets of San Francisco tracking down drug pushers for the Narcotics Bureau. Sometimes after a tough day on the beat he invited his narc buddies up to one of the safehouses for a little "R & R." Occasionally they unzipped their inhibitions and partied on the premises—much to the chagrin of the neighbors, who began to complain about men with guns in shoulder straps chasing after women in various states of undress. Needless to say, there was always plenty of dope around, and the feds sampled everything from hashish to LSD. "So far as I'm concerned," White later told an associate, " 'clear thinking' was non-existent while under the influence of any of these drugs. I did feel at times like I was having a 'mind-expanding experience' but this vanished like a dream immediately after the session." White had quite a scene going for a while. By day he fought to keep drugs out of circulation, and by night he dispensed them to strangers. Not everyone was cut out for this kind of schizophrenic lifestyle, and White often relied on the bottle to reconcile the two extremes. But there were still moments when his Jekyll-and-Hyde routine got the best of him. One night a friend who had helped install bugging equipment for the CIA stopped by the safehouse only to find the roly-poly narcotics officer slumped in front of a full-length mirror. White had just finished polishing off a half gallon of Gibson's. There he sat, with gun in hand, shooting wax slugs at his own reflection. The safehouse experiments continued without interruption until 1963, when CIA inspector general John Earman accidentally stumbled across the clandestine testing program during a routine inspection of TSS operations. Only a handful of CIA agents outside Technical Services knew about the testing of LSD on unwitting subjects, and Earman took Richard Helms, the prime instigator of MK-ULTRA, to task for not fully briefing the new CIA director, John J. McCone. Although McCone had been handpicked by President Kennedy to replace Allen Dulles as the dean of American intelligence, Helms apparently had his own ideas about who was running the CIA.

Earman had grave misgivings about MK-ULTRA and he prepared a twenty-four-page report that included a comprehensive overview of the drug and mind control projects. In a cover letter to McCone he noted that the "concepts involved in manipulating human behavior are found by many people within and outside the Agency to be distasteful and unethical." But the harshest criticism was reserved for the safehouse experiments, which, in his words, placed "the rights and interests of U.S. citizens in jeopardy." Earman stated that LSD had been tested on "individuals at all social levels, high and low, native American and foreign." Numerous subjects had become ill, and some required hospitalization for days or weeks at a time. Moreover, the sophomoric procedures employed during the safehouse sessions raised serious questions about the validity of the data provided by White, who was hardly a qualified scientist. As Earman pointed out, the CIA had no way of knowing whether White was fudging the results to suit his own ends. Earman recommended a freeze on unwitting drug tests until the matter was fully considered at the highest level of the CIA. But Helms, then deputy director for covert operations (the number two position within the Agency), defended the program. In a memo dated November 9, 1964, he warned that the CIA's "positive operational capacity to use drugs is diminishing owing to a lack of realistic testing," and he called for a resumption of the safehouse experiments. While admitting that he had "no answer to the moral issue," Helms argued that such tests were necessary "to keep up with Soviet advances in this field." This Cold War refrain had a familiar ring. Yet only a few months earlier Helms had sung a different tune when J. Lee Rankin, chief counsel of the Warren Commission investigating the Kennedy assassination, asked him to report on Soviet mind control initiatives. Helms stated his views in a document dated June 26, 1964: "Soviet research in the pharmacological agents producing behavioral effects has consistently lagged five years behind Western research [emphasis added]." Furthermore, he confidently asserted that the Russians did not have "any singular, new potent drugs... to force a course of action on an individual." The bureaucratic wrangling at CIA headquarters didn't seem to bother George Hunter White, who kept on sending vouchers for "unorthodox expenses" to Dr. Sidney Gottlieb. No definitive record exists as to when the unwitting acid tests were terminated, but it appears that White and the CIA parted ways when he retired from the Narcotics Bureau in 1966. Afterwards White reflected upon his service for the Agency in a letter to Gottlieb: "I was a very minor missionary, actually a heretic, but I toiled wholeheartedly in the vineyards because it was fun, fun, fun. Where else could a red-blooded American boy lie, kill, cheat, steal, rape, and pillage with the sanction and blessing of the All-Highest?" By this time the CIA had developed a "stable of drugs," including LSD, that were used in covert operations. The decision to employ LSD on an operational basis was handled through a special committee that reported directly to Richard Helms, who characterized the drug as "dynamite" and asked to be "advised at all times when it was intended for use." A favorite plan involved slipping "P-1" (the code name for LSD when used operationally) to socialist or left-leaning politicians in foreign countries so that they would babble incoherently and discredit themselves in public.[11]

But before the agency's shady history of LSD became public, they were still searching for ways to utilize its full power—handing the drug out to a host of doctors and scientists that would become modern day mad scientists creating psychedelic Frankenstein's.

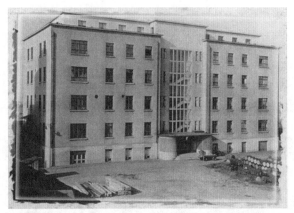

Old Sandoz Laboratory, Since Demolished (*Hoffman.org*)

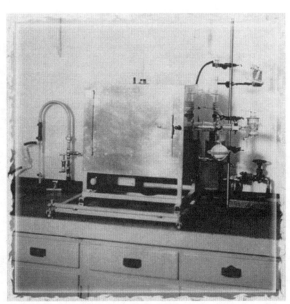

Equipment for the Bromination of LSD in Dr. Hofmann's Laboratory
(*Hoffman.org*)

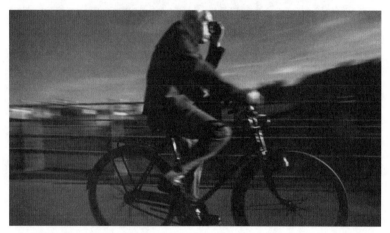

Albert Hofmann's trippy bicycle ride (*Hoffman.org*)

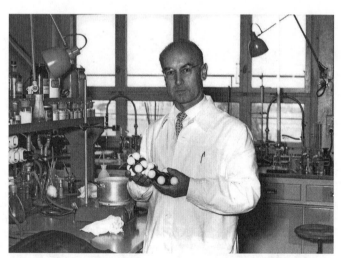

Albert Hofmann's accidental discovery of LSD's effects led to it being
used in psychiatry (*Bhekisisa*)

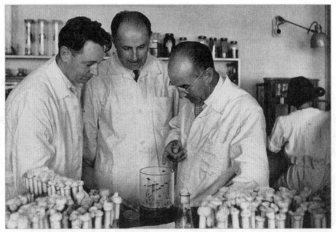

Hofmann, right, cultivates mushrooms (*NY Times*)

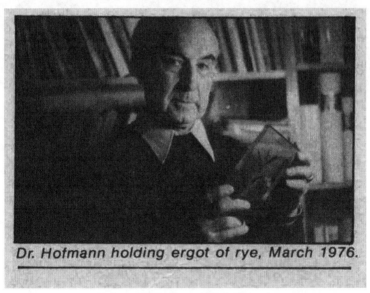

Dr. Hofmann holding ergot of rye, March 1976.

Albert Hofmann (*High Times*)

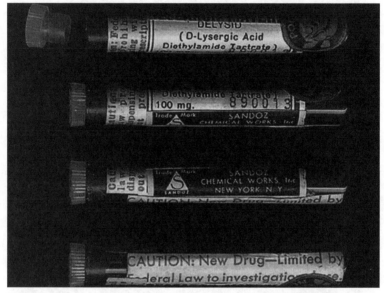

Sandoz Chemical Works antique vials (*Pinterest*)

Chapter Three

Daytrippers:
The CIA's Mad LSD Scientists

*Psychedelics are illegal not because a loving government
is concerned that you may jump out of a third story
window. Psychedelics are illegal because they dissolve
opinion structures and culturally laid down models of
behavior and information processing. They open you up to
the possibility that everything you know is wrong.*
—Terence McKenna

After years of searching, the agency felt they were finally on the verge of finding the end-all, be-all of truth serums thanks to LSD. With the substance, the cloak-and-dagger trade would never be the same but the CIA ran into problems after realizing that LSD wasn't your typical truth serum, as most test subjects opted to unlock the secrets of the universe rather than to spew off secrets of the state. Accurate and beneficial information was increasingly harder to come by as LSD seemed to heighten anxiety and cause patients to temporally lose touch with reality. Bouts of intense time distortion, paranoid meltdowns and bizarre hallucinations caused by LSD proved more of a nuisance than help during the interrogation process. What if the spy realized that he had been drugged? Certainly, if they had been slipped a mickey of LSD it wouldn't take but a few hours to realize that something was definitely wrong, in which case they would most likely get suspicious and clam up. But even more precarious situations could erupt during an interrogation, what if the subject experienced delusions of grandeur and transcendental omnipotence? An entire operation could backfire if the suspects suddenly became convinced of their sudden Superman-esque possibilities. Then there were the overoptimistic views of LSD causing amnesia in interrogation subjects. It didn't work most of the time as test subjects experienced memory distortion to certain degrees without actually going blank, recalling most of their trips while knowing that something extraordinary was indeed happening to them. But the CIA scientists kept testing away, convinced that LSD could still be the truth serum they had hoped it would be even though the unusual substance failed to live up to its original expectations. They had to shift gears and reassess the future potential of LSD,\; if the drug wasn't a reliable truth serum, then what else could it be?

CIA researchers were at a loss to figure out what this new chemical could be used for, as LSD was light years beyond any psychedelic compound they knew about. CIA scientists marveled at how the colorless, odorless, and tasteless drug could have such a mystifying effect with only minute quantities being administered. The problem was that not everyone reacted in the same manner when high on LSD and that it was hard to predict the response. On some occasions the drug caused the subjects to spew an avalanche of information, but these were rare occurrences as LSD usually overwhelmed them to the point of making the interrogation process a comedic skit. The drug itself was bipolar as it caused mood swings from full blown panic to boundless joys of emotional bliss. Scientists scratched their heads while trying to figure out how one drug could produce such a wide range of contradictory reactions. As research continued, the mystery surrounding LSD became more perplexing as the agency decided that it could be used as an anti-interrogation substance, postulating that the drug could serve in a sort of suicide pill scenario where agents would drown the drug before falling into enemy hands. The LSD would provide a counter measure for the captured spy who would most likely spew steady streams of Archer-style spy babble gibberish. But what if the agent had the opposite reaction and told the truth about his mission!

The CIA's top scientists didn't know what to make of LSD. First they thought it was a truth serum, then a lie serum, and all the while they were trying to figure out just how to use it, there was the worry that the Russian and Chinese commies were also experimenting with the drug as an espionage weapon. The Office of Scientific Intelligence was well aware that ergot was a commercial product in numerous Eastern Bloc countries and although it hadn't yet hit the Russian market, ergot was known to be a common fungus throughout the country. Surely the Soviets were aware of LSD, ergot's mind blowing cousin, as it had already been mentioned in scientific journals as early as 1947. Perhaps the Russians were stockpiling raw ergot with the hopes of doing their own LSD mind control experiments? This range of thinking certainly didn't escape the CIA who were worried that it might be true. John Gittlinger, one of the CIA's leading Cold War psychologists, was convinced they were experimenting with LSD even though he had never seen any proof of it; despite this the company wasn't taking any chances. But it seems that the Soviets weren't conducting any psychedelic experiments that we know of at the time. Dozens of experiments involving the psychedelic drug were carried out in Communist Bulgaria from 1962 to 1968 by Bulgarian psychiatrist Marina Boyadjieva, but that's way after the CIA got involved. There were more than 140 Bulgarian acid tests that studied the usual arrangement of human guinea pigs like artists, prisoners and mentally ill patients. Bulgaria was a pretty lame place in the early years of the Cold War—recreational drugs were unheard of—western music was illegal and the thought of reaching innerspace via LSD was something one might read in a hippie comic book somewhere in Manhattan, certainly not obtainable way out in Bulgaria. But experimental treatments of psychosis in mentally healthy people was a hot topic in pharmacology and psychiatry circles after World War II. Professor Boyadjieva was lucky enough to acquire a small batch of LSD when she was a research assistant at the Department of Psychiatry at the Medical University of Sofia, in Bulgaria. "In 1961, I met a Sandoz representative by the name of Mr. Burge. He told me they had LSD in doses of 0.025 mg. This was the so-called LSD-25," recalled Boyadjieva. "In the beginning, I asked for a box of 50 ampoules, and later Mr. Burge brought me more. I administered refined LSD in small doses to the volunteers. It was a wholly organic substance. Clear as a teardrop!"[1]

Doing LSD experiments at the Multiprofile Hospital for Active Treatment in Neurology and Psychiatry–St. Naum, in the Bulgarian capital of Sofia, the volunteers would either ingest a sugar-coated tablet of Delysid containing 0.025 mg of LSD, or get injected with 100 micrograms of the drug. There was always a nurse on standby with a shot of 50 mg of the antipsychotic drug Chlorpromazine just in case the subjects started freaking out. Soon word of Boyadjieva's activities came to the attention of the army, which promptly paid a visit. "The Cold War was at its peak. Apparently our military had heard some disconcerting things about the LSD experiments conducted in the West at that time, they were interested if the drug could be used as a weapon of mass destruction or a truth serum. They literally asked me: "Can they [the West] make us go crazy with it?"[2]

She then signed a confidentiality agreement with the army and began conducting experiments on soldiers, injecting them with 25 micrograms of LSD while in the presence of a colonel and a military psychiatrist. The secret LSD experiments were filmed by the military, which confiscated all reports concerning Boyadjieva's tests. She never heard from the army officials again, and the footage of her LSD experiments with the Bulgarian army has yet to resurface. Bulgaria wasn't the only country behind the Iron Curtain interested in LSD experiments back then. The young Czech doctor Stanislav Grof began conducting clinical experiments with LSD in 1958 at the Prague Psychiatric Research Institute. "If I am the father of LSD," Hofmann, the drug's inventor, famously said, "Stan Grof is the godfather." Another Czech physician, Dr. Milan Hausner, conducted over 6,000 LSD sessions between 1956 and 1974 during the Czech army's research into psychedelic weapons of war.

If an American spy was dosed by commies he better be able to recognize it, so almost all spies in the early 50s were given LSD so the company could gauge their anxieties and abilities while tripping. More exposure to the drug guaranteed that operatives were in a better position to handle the experience and wouldn't freak out while continuing their mission under the hazy gauze of LSD. CIA documents referred to some of the more spiritually awakened agents as "enlightened operatives"[3], or those who experienced the spiritual door-opening effect that LSD can lead to. But most agents and CIA trainee volunteers that were administered the drug were anxiety-riddled basket cases that couldn't pass the acid test and were left to work in the far less interesting fields of the agency. With full approval from the CIA's Medical Office, and shielded by Project ARTICHOKE, the agency spent at least three full years giving their agents, volunteers and kidnapped mental patients LSD without the public knowing anything about it. Internal CIA documents revealed that the agency's LSD experiments reignited an interest in ESP and other phenomena rooted in altered states of consciousness:

The CIA's interest in parapsychology dates back to the late 1940s. A handwritten memo of the period suggests that "hypnotists and telepathists" be contacted as professional consultants on an exploratory basis, but this proposal was initially rejected. It was not until 1952, after the CIA got heavily involved with LSD, that the Agency began funding ESP research. While parapsychology has long been ridiculed by the scientific establishment, the CIA seriously entertained the notion that such phenomena might be highly significant for the spy trade. The Agency hypothesized that if a number of people in the US were found to have a high ESP capacity, their talent could be assigned to specific intelligence problems. In 1952 the CIA initiated an extensive program involving "the search for and development of exceptionally gifted individuals who can approximate perfect success in ESP performance." The Office of Security, which ran the ARTICHOKE project, was urged to follow "all leads on individuals reported to have true clairvoyant powers" so as to be able to subject their claims to "rigorous scientific investigation." Along this line the CIA began infiltrating séances and occult gatherings. A memo dated April 9, 1953, refers to a domestic—and therefore illegal—operation that required the "planting of a very specialized observer" at a séance in order to obtain "a broad surveillance of all individuals attending the meetings." At the outset of the CIA's behavior control endeavors the main emphasis was on speech-inducing drugs. But when acid entered the scene, the entire program assumed a more aggressive posture. The CIA's turned-on strategists came to believe that mind control techniques could be applied to a wide range of operations above and beyond the strict category of "special interrogation." It was almost as if LSD blew the Agency's collective mind-set—or was it mind-rut? With acid acting as a catalyst, the whole idea of what could be done with a drug or drugs in general, was suddenly transformed. Soon a perfect compound was envisioned for every conceivable circumstance: there would be smart shots, memory erasers, "anti vitamins," knock-out drops, "aphrodisiacs for operational use," drugs that caused "headache clusters" or uncontrollable twitching, drugs that could induce cancer, a stroke or a heart attack without leaving a trace as to the source of the ailment. There were chemicals to make a drunk man sober and a sober man as drunk as a fish. Even a "recruitment pill" was contemplated. What's more, according to a document dated May 5, 1955, the CIA placed a high priority on the development of a drug "which will produce 'pure euphoria' with no subsequent letdown." This is not to suggest that the CIA had given up on LSD. On the contrary, after grappling with the drug for a number of years, the Agency devised new methods of interrogation based on the "far-out" possibilities of this mind-altering substance. When employed as a third-degree tactic, acid enabled the CIA to approach a hostile subject with a great deal of leverage. CIA operatives realized that intense mental confusion could be produced by deliberately attacking a person along psychological lines. Of all the chemicals that caused mental derangement, none was as powerful as LSD. Acid not only made people extremely anxious, it also broke down the character defenses for handling anxiety. A skillful interrogator could exploit this vulnerability by threatening to keep an unwitting subject in a tripped-out state indefinitely unless he spilled the beans. This tactic often proved successful where others had failed.[4]

LSD was employed as an interrogation tool for at least a decade, and it sometimes served as a catalyst for a crew of psychics the agency employed to develop their powers of ESP. If LSD somehow made psychics more psychic, then the agency was for sure going to find out by plying them with the drug and assigning them missions to attend occult gatherings, séances and even remote viewing sessions where they hoped they could see through walls and gather information from miles away. The CIA even conducted experiments that tried to contact dead agents as part of a larger effort to develop psychic powers for various clairvoyant related intelligence missions. Recently declassified CIA files have revealed that the company used psychics to spy on Iran and they even held the famous clairvoyant Uri Geller hostage while they ran a series of mind blowing tests on him. The Stargate Program was aimed at finding out whether humans could use psychic powers as weapons or spy tools like they were X-Men mutants or something. During the program the agency carried out a set of secret psychic experiments on Uri Geller and were shocked when he accurately predicted an agent's drawing from the next room over.[5] It turns out that Geller wasn't only adept at bending spoons, he could also bend minds. The Israeli was taken to the Stanford Research Institute to have his psychic abilities investigated. He passed with flying colors as the CIA researchers concluded that, "Uri, demonstrated his paranormal perceptual ability in a convincing and unambiguous manner."[6] Uri, perhaps history's most famous psychic spy has been known to work for both the CIA and the Mossad. It's curious to note that he has never admitted to taking LSD; surely the company would be interested in giving the world's greatest psychic a hit of the drug just to see what would happen.

Spoon-bending aside, the CIA was in a constant hunt for American laboratories capable of handling these secret LSD experiments, as only a handful of scientists at the time were engaging in hallucinogenic psychedelic research. There was little to no private or public support for this new field of experimental psychedelic psychiatry, so, to no one's surprise, the first serious investigations of LSD came under the cloak and dagger skullduggery of the CIA. But with a sizable treasure chest at their disposal, the agency looked to boost the careers and pocketbooks of scientists daring enough to participate in this great new scientific unknown. Overnight, a whole new market for grants in LSD and psychedelic research sprang into being as money started gushing through CIA-linked fronts like the Geschickter Fund for Medical Research, the Society for the Study of Human Ecology, and the Josiah Macy, Jr. Foundation among others.

The CIA also found out that Doctors Max Rinkel and Robert Hyde were the first people to bring LSD to the United States in 1949, and that Rinkel had the honor of taking the first acid trip in the West. The good doctors organized an LSD study at the Boston Psychopathic

Institute, a pioneering mental health clinic affiliated with Harvard University, and tested the drug on over a hundred volunteers nearly three years before the CIA began funding their experiments. Rinkel was the first to recognize the potential therapeutic breakthroughs LSD could make as certain mental disorders could be studied objectively in a controlled environment. Dr. Paul Hoch, a prominent psychiatrist and future CIA beneficiary, agreed with Rinkel as they both offered a positive outlook on LSD to the panel at an annual meeting of the American Psychiatric Association in 1951 (Hoch would change his tune later, as we have seen):

> Hoch reported that the symptoms produced by LSD, mescaline and related drugs were similar to those of schizophrenia: intensity of color perception, hallucinations, depersonalization, intense anxiety, paranoia, and in some cases catatonic manifestations. As Hoch put it, "LSD and Mescaline disorganize the psychic integration of the individual." He believed that the medical profession was fortunate to have access to these substances, for now it would be possible to reconstruct temporary or "model" psychoses in the laboratory. LSD was considered an exceptional research tool in that the subject could provide a detailed description of his experience while he was under the influence of the drug. It was hoped that careful analysis of these data would shed new light on schizophrenia and other enigmatic mental diseases. Hoch's landmark thesis—that LSD was a "psychotomimetic" or "madness-mimicking" agent—caused a sensation in scientific circles and led to several important and stimulating theories regarding the biochemical basis of schizophrenia. This in turn sparked an upsurge of interest in brain chemistry and opened new vistas in the field of experimental psychiatry. In light of the extremely high potency of LSD, it seemed completely plausible that infinitesimal traces of a psychoactive substance produced through metabolic dysfunction by the human organism might cause psychotic disturbances. Conversely, attempts to alleviate a "lysergic psychosis" might point the way toward curing schizophrenia and other forms of mental

illness. While the miracle cure never panned out, it is worth noting that Thorazine was found to mollify an LSD reaction and subsequently became a standard drug for controlling patients in mental asylums and prisons. As it turned out, the model psychosis concept dovetailed particularly well with the secret schemes of the CIA, which also viewed LSD in terms of its ability to blow minds and make people crazy. Thus it is not surprising that the CIA chose to invest in men like Rinkel and Hoch. Most scientists were flattered by the government's interest in their research, and they were eager to assist the CIA in its attempt to unravel the riddle of LSD. This was, after all, the Cold War, and one did not have to be a blue-ribbon hawk or a hard liner to work in tandem with American intelligence.[7]

This was the case when the CIA approached the psychiatrist Dr. Nick Bercel, who maintained a private practice in Los Angeles and was one of the first people to use LSD as a therapeutic tool on his patients. But what the CIA wanted to know wasn't the progress his patients might be making, but what would happen if the Russians spiked the city's water supply with LSD. *The Fortean Times* expounds:

> The psychedelic water saga arose at the height of the Cold War in 1953, when the intelligence agency approached Dr. Nick Bercel, a Los Angeles psychiatrist working with LSD in a psychotherapeutic context. After querying him on the possible consequences if the Russians were to put LSD in the water supply of a large American city, the spooks demanded Bercel calculate how much LSD would be needed to dose Los Angeles's water supply with acid. Bercel dissolved some LSD in a glass of chlorinated water, which promptly neutralized the psychedelic, leading him to tell the CIA the idea was not worth pursuing. The spooks were unconvinced, allegedly designing another version of LSD that was not neutralized by chlorine. Yet although the experiment had failed, the idea that LSD could be used to mass-dose the population had been created—and even

though scientific opinion was against it, the notion was just too powerful to give up and started to take on a life of its own. Dr. Jim Ketchum was involved in the US Army's program for testing the military effectiveness of a whole range of psychedelic chemicals. He entered his office as Department Chief one Monday morning in 1969 and found a black steel barrel, a bit like an oil drum, in the corner. The military does not always explain everything, and Dr. Ketchum assumed there was a good reason for this unusual addition to the furniture. However, after a couple of days he became curious. He waited until everyone else in the building had gone home one evening and opened the lid. The barrel was filled with sealed glass canisters "like cookie jars". He took one out to inspect it; the label indicated that the jar contained three pounds of pure EA 1729. This wouldn't mean much to most people, but to anyone working in this field the code was instantly familiar. Substances were given EA designations from the Army's Edgewood Arsenal; EA 1729 is the military designation for LSD. The other glass canisters were the same, perhaps 14 of them in all. This was enough acid for several hundred million doses with, Ketchum estimated, a street value of over a billion dollars. Some wild ideas about what to do next flitted through his mind, but in the event he simply sealed the barrel up again. By the Friday morning it had vanished as mysteriously as it arrived.[8]

It's almost shocking that the CIA never false flagged an entire city by dropping a massive dose of LSD in the water supply. This is exactly how the both Joker and the Scarecrow threatened to turn on the citizens of Gotham City before Batman foiled their dastardly plot. To the CIA, the idea of spiking a town's water supply was a foregone conclusion; hell if they couldn't spike your water they'd figure out some other wacko way to get LSD in your system as stated in a declassified document:

If the concept of contaminating a city's water supply seems, or in actual fact, is found to be far-fetched (this is by no means certain), there is still the possibility of contaminating, say, the water supply of a bomber base or, more easily still, that of a battleship.... Our current work contains the strong suggestion that LSD-25 will produce hysteria (unaccountable laughing, anxiety, terror).... It requires little imagination to realize what the consequences might be if a battleship's crew were so affected.[9]

The CIA backed off from working with Bercel, but they continued to monitor his research reports concerning LSD in various medical journals. Bercel did many experiments giving LSD to animals, discovering that spiders tended to spin perfectly symmetrical webs and that cats were kinda spooked by mice. Footage of Bercel conducting an LSD experiment on the artist William Millarc can be seen on Youtube. Officially titled "Schizophrenic Model Psychosis Induced by Lysergic Acid Diethylamide (LSD)" the startling film was dug up from the National Archives and documents an LSD test at the University of California as supervised by Dr. Bercel. The subject was artist William Millarc who was given a dose of LSD-25 and then interviewed while tripping. He seemed to enjoy the trip as he noted the psychedelic colors of the swaying carpet with a smile on his face. A few years later he would commit suicide with the hope that his paintings would end up more valuable. They didn't. From the *EL Paso Herald-Post*, April 29, 1957:

A despondent, debt-haunted artist, from Glendale, Calif., committed suicide and left a wry note saying that perhaps his death would make his paintings more valuable, police said today. William Millarc, 37, shot himself in the head Saturday and left a note that read: "My paintings don't meet the bills. Maybe my death will make them valuable enough." Officers said Millarc killed himself with a .38 caliber pistol he brought with him to a dinner party at the home of friends. His wife, Heydee, 31, said Millarc was, "ever worried" about pending bills he didn't have the money to pay. His paintings had been shown at local art galleries and at the county museum and some of his oils won high critical praise in 1951, yet Millarc had been forced to work as an art instructor to make a living.[10]

Meanwhile the CIA's interest in LSD continued as they supervised research carried out by Dr. Louis Jolyon West, chairman of the Department of Psychiatry at the University of Oklahoma and master of mind control. He even injected a massive dose of LSD into an elephant once but the animal just keeled over and remained in a motionless acid trip stupor until the poor thing died from a combination of drugs meant to save him. Dr. West was a high-ranking CIA psychiatrist who once proposed to experiment on the brains of blacks and Latino prisoners in a secret psychiatric unit set up at an abandoned missile silo in the hills near UCLA. Dr. West believed that, "in some patients, outbursts of uncontrolled rage have definitely been linked to abnormal electrical activity in deeply buried areas of the brain... For many years, neurologists have measured the electrical activity of the brain with electrodes attached to the scalp... Now by implanting tiny electrodes deep within the brain, electrical activity can be followed in areas that cannot be measured from the surface of the scalp... It is even possible to record bioelectrical changes in the brains of freely moving subjects, through the use of remote monitoring techniques."[11]

Dr. West's racist psychiatric experiment wouldn't be allowed to get off the ground but he still maintained top secret clearance and a high spot on the ladder when it came to position within the scientific circles of MK-ULTRA. LSD research continued to confound the CIA as they discovered that LSD lodged primarily in the areas of the liver, spleen, and kidneys, and only less than .02% of the original dose entered the brain. Even stranger was the fact that the drug remained there for twenty minutes without effect until the LSD had disappeared from the central nervous system entirely. Scientists still couldn't figure out exactly why the drug had such a dramatic effect on the mind and why each trip differed upon various personalities. They were still trying to figure out the maximum dosage before fatality and if there was some sort of antidote to counter the effects of the drug:

Some of these questions overlapped with legitimate medical concerns, and researchers on CIA stipends published unclassified versions of their work in prestigious scientific periodicals. But these accounts omitted secret data given to the CIA on how LSD affected "operationally pertinent categories" such as disturbance of memory, alteration of sex patterns, eliciting information, increasing suggestibility, and creating emotional dependence. The CIA was particularly interested in psychiatric reports suggesting that LSD could break down familiar behavior patterns, for this raised the possibility of reprogramming or brainwashing. If LSD temporarily altered a person's view of the world and suspended his belief system, CIA doctors surmised, then perhaps Russian spies could be cajoled into switching loyalties while they were tripping...LSD would be employed to provoke a reality shift, to break someone down and tame him, to find a locus of anonymity and leave a mark there forever. To explore the feasibility of this approach, the Agency turned to Dr. Ewen Cameron, a respected psychiatrist who served as president of the Canadian, the American, and the World Psychiatric Associations before his death in 1967.[12]

With financial help from the CIA, Cameron developed a bizarre method for treating schizophrenia with a combination of sleep and electroshock therapy under the influence of LSD. The mad scientist would confine his heavily sedated patients to sleeping rooms where tape recorded messages and sounds played over a quarter of a million times from speakers under their pillows. Talk about a bad trip. Cameron's methods were later discredited, and nine of his former patients later sued the American government for a million dollars each, claiming they never agreed to participate in scientific LSD experiments overseen by the CIA. Even though the agency had violated the Nuremberg Code of medical ethics by sponsoring experiments on unwitting subjects, they hardly seemed to care and continued on conducting business as usual.

Like the project undertaken at the Addiction Research Center of the US Public Health Service Hospital in Lexington, Kentucky a place where they had all heroin addict "patients" they could ever dream of. The patients had no way of knowing they were soon to

Liquid Conspiracy 2

be the guinea pigs from one of fifteen penal and mental institutions utilized by the CIA in covert drug development programs. The agency concealed its role in the program by enlisting the aid of the National Institutes of Mental Health (NIMH), the conduit that channeled the funds to Dr. Harris Isbell, a research scientist happy to be working for the CIA. Isbell received a variety of hallucinogens including LSD and soon began enticing street junkies to commit to Lexington where they would get all the heroin and morphine needed in return for volunteering in Isbell's wacky LSD experiments. CIA documents described experiments conducted by Isbell in which certain patients were given LSD for more than seventy-five consecutive days in a quest to judge the drug's tolerance. About 95% of the patients were impoverished black men, who were given double, triple and quadruple doses of LSD and psilocybin compounds from magic mushrooms. But lengthy laugh attacks and prolonged fantastic acid trips did little to further the agency's understanding of psychedelics:

>In addition to his role as a research scientist, Dr. Isbell served as a go-between for the CIA in its attempt to obtain drug samples from European pharmaceutical concerns which assumed they were providing "medicine" to a US Public Health official. The CIA in turn acted as a research coordinator, passing information, tips, and leads to Isbell and its other contract employees so that they could keep abreast of each other's progress; when a new discovery was made, the CIA would often ask another researcher to conduct a follow-up study for confirmation. One scientist whose work was coordinated with Isbell's in such a manner was Dr. Carl Pfeiffer, a noted pharmacologist from Princeton who tested LSD on inmates at the federal prison in Atlanta and the Bordentown Reformatory in New Jersey. Isbell, Pfeiffer, Cameron, West, and Hoch—all were part of a network of doctors and scientists who gathered intelligence for the CIA. Through these scholar-informants the agency stayed on top of the latest developments within the "aboveground" LSD scene, which expanded rapidly during the Cold War. By the mid-1950s numerous independent investigators had undertaken hallucinogenic drug studies, and the CIA was

determined not to let the slightest detail escape its grasp. In a communiqué dated May 26, 1954, the agency ordered all domestic field offices in the United States to monitor scientists engaged in LSD research. People of interest, the memo explained, "will most probably be found in biochemistry departments of universities, mental hospitals, private psychiatric practice…. We do ask that you remember their importance and report their work when it comes to your attention." The CIA also expended considerable effort to monitor the latest developments in LSD research on a worldwide scale. Drug specialists funded by the Agency made periodic trips to Europe to confer with scientists and representatives of various pharmaceutical concerns, including, of course, Sandoz Laboratories. Initially the Swiss firm provided LSD to investigators all over the world free of charge, in exchange for full access to their research data. (CIA researchers did not comply with this stipulation.) By 1953 Sandoz had decided to deal directly with the US Food and Drug Administration (FDA), which assumed a supervisory role in distributing LSD to American investigators from then on. It was a superb arrangement as far as the CIA was concerned, for the FDA went out of its way to assist the secret drug program. With the FDA as its junior partner, the CIA not only had ready access to supplies of LSD (which Sandoz marketed for a while under the brand name Delysid) but also was able to keep a close eye on independent researchers in the United States. The CIA would have been content to let the FDA act as an intermediary in its dealings with Sandoz, but business as usual was suspended when the agency learned of an offer that could not be refused. Prompted by reports that large quantities of the drug were suddenly available, top-level CIA officials authorized the purchase of ten kilos of LSD from Sandoz at an estimated price of $240,000 enough for a staggering one hundred million doses. A document dated November 16, 1953 characterized the pending transaction as a "risky operation," but CIA officials felt it was necessary, if only to preclude any attempt the Communists might make to get their hands on the drug. What the CIA intended to do with such an incredible stash of acid was never made clear. The CIA later found out that Sandoz had never produced LSD in quantities even remotely resembling ten kilograms. Apparently only ten milligrams were for sale, but a CIA contact in Switzerland mistook for a milligram (.001 grams) for a kilogram, 1000 grams, which would explain the huge discrepancy. Nevertheless, Sandoz officials were pleased by the CIA's interest in their product, and the two organizations struck up a cooperative relationship.[13]

With an ironclad arrangement and full disclosure from Arthur Stoll, president of Sandoz, the CIA locked down the future of LSD by securing a monopoly on the drug. Any future information about who bought the drug or where it was being shipped was immediately relayed to the CIA. But the agency wasn't comfortable with having to depend on a foreign company all the way in Switzerland for supplies of a substance considered to be the Holy Grail when it came to a possible mind control weapon/truth serum—so they asked the Eli Lilly Company to try to synthesize a batch of all-American acid. By the summer of 1954, the scientists at the Lilly laboratory in Indianapolis had succeeded in breaking the secret formula held by Sandoz and informed the CIA that in a matter of months their American-made LSD would be available by the ton. This was good news as more scientists were given the drug to experiment with.

Another CIA mad scientist who rented his services to both the agency and the military was Dr. Robert Heath of Tulane University. Heath was a hands-on sort of fellow as he and his colleagues administered LSD to people while subjecting them to electronic brain stimulation therapy via electrode implant. Not a good trip. But Heath wasn't interested in the army's search for a truth serum, he was more interested in curing gay people by frying their brains. Heath's gay cure experiments have largely been written out of scientific history, and his claims of curing homosexuality by implanting electrodes into the pleasure center of the brain dismissed. But Heath was a suave scientist-hero, a Cary Grant lookalike in a white lab coat. "He looked like a god—and carried himself like one," his former colleague Marilyn Skinner reminisced. Besides being a top CIA scientist he was board certified in both psychiatry and neurology and a qualified psychoanalyst:

He could treat a patient, diagnose a mental illness, read an EEG and dash off a paper, all before heading off to the country club for a round of golf. Born in 1915 in Pittsburgh, Heath trained as a neurologist, before being drafted into service as a military psychiatrist in World War II. He rapidly aligned himself with the new breed of biological psychiatrists—scientists who argued that what were traditionally thought of as diseases of the mind were often actually diseases of the brain and could therefore be cured through surgery, not therapy. There was already some obvious evidence for this, in the shape of the way that patients' behaviour changed after prefrontal lobotomy. This was the most widespread form of what was known as psychosurgery—the surgical treatment of mental illness. Yet even though the procedure, which involved chopping away the connections to much of the brain's frontal lobe, was growing in popularity, Heath and his colleagues at Columbia University rightly viewed it as crude and ineffective. They decided to compare it with a much less invasive alternative, which they called topectomy: this involved targeting and removing specific areas of the cortex, in order to avoid wider damage to the brain. Among these were his efforts to treat gay men by turning "repugnant feelings... toward the opposite sex" into pleasurable ones— and similar work on "frigid women." He experimented with dripping drugs deep into the brain down tiny pipes called cannulae, targeting the same regions as his electrodes. He tested a 'brainwashing' drug called bulbocapnine for the CIA, on both animals and (although he denied it for decades) on a human prisoner, as a small part of the vast and largely illegal 'MK-ULTRA' programme to explore the limits and limitations of the American body. He talked a suicidal patient down from a roof. He injected horseradish peroxidase into the brain to see how it carried chemicals. He gave a talk to the Army on electrical stimulation of the brain, after which his department was contracted to test

69

psychoactive drugs on prisoners: the resulting paper, from 1957, is as macabre and gripping as the studies involving B-19, complete with detailed descriptions of the patients' behaviour and hallucinations.[14]

Heath was a mad scientist if there ever was one. In 1995, Claudia Mullen testified before Congress that Heath treated her as a child patient, and subjected her to all kinds of unethical practices before handing her over to the CIA, where she was used as a sex slave. The army had their own mad LSD scientists conducting extensive in-house studies at Fort Bragg, North Carolina, for seeing just how well soldiers would fare during war games while high on acid. Small military units were given LSD (code-named EA 1729), and asked to perform various operational exercises, including tank driving, radarscope reading, antiaircraft drills and engineering surveys, etc. The soldiers were filmed and the footage was later shown to members of Congress to demonstrate the disruptive influence of psychedelics:

> Concerned that LSD might one day be used covertly against an American military unit, certain officials suggested that every Chemical Corps officer should be familiar with the effects of the drug, if only as a precautionary measure. Accordingly nearly two hundred officers assigned to the Chemical Corps school at Fort McClellan, Alabama, were given acid as a supplement to their regular training program. Some staff members even tried to teach classes while tripping. Additional tests were carried out at the Aberdeen Proving Ground in Maryland; Fort Benning, Georgia; Fort Leavenworth, Kansas; Dugway Proving Ground, Utah; and in various European and Pacific stations. Soldiers at Edgewood Arsenal were given LSD and confined to sensory deprivation chambers; then they were subjected to hostile questioning by intelligence officers. An army report concludes that an "interrogator of limited experience could compel a subject to compromise himself and to sign documents which could place him in jeopardy." With a stronger dose "a state of fear and anxiety could be induced where the subject could

be compelled to trade his cooperation for a guarantee of return to normalcy." Shortly thereafter the military began using LSD as an interrogation weapon on an operational basis, just as the CIA had been doing for years. An army memo dated September 6, 1961, discussed the interrogation procedure: "Stressing techniques employed included silent treatment before or after EA 1729 administration, sustained conventional interrogation prior to EA 1729 interrogation, deprivation of food, drink, sleep or bodily evacuation, sustained isolation prior to EA 1729 administration, hotcold switches in approach, duress 'pitches,' verbal degradation and bodily discomfort, or dramatized threats to subject's life or mental health." Documents pertaining to Operation DERBY HAT indicate that an army Special Purpose Team trained in LSD interrogations initiated a series of field tests in the Far East beginning in August 1962. Seven individuals were questioned; all were foreign nationals who had been implicated in drug smuggling or espionage activities, and in each case the EA-I729 technique produced information that had not been obtained through other means. One subject vomited three times and stated that he "wanted to die" after the Special Purpose Team gave him LSD; his reaction was characterized as "moderate." Another went into shock and remained semiconscious for nearly an hour after receiving triple the dosage normally used in these sessions. When he came to, the Special Purpose Team propped him up in a chair and tried to question him, but the subject kept collapsing and hitting his head on the table, oblivious to the pain. A few hours later he started to talk. "The subject often voiced an anticommunist line," an army report noted, "and begged to be spared the torture he was receiving. In this confused state he even asked to be killed in order to alleviate his suffering."[15]

By the time acid hit the streets, nearly 1,500 military personnel had served as guinea pigs in secret LSD experiments conducted by the US Army Chemical Corps, not to mention the others exposed from the supply that some soldiers swiped from the Edgewood

Arsenal. Some of these soldiers had their first "trip" (originally coined by army scientists to describe an LSD session) at spiked punch bowl mess parties. Army Major General Creasy wanted large-scale public drills of psychochemical weapons, "to test to see what would happen in subways, for example, when a cloud was laid down on a city. It was denied on reasons that always seemed a little absurd to me." But army scientists found out that LSD was more effective by ingestion than by cloud-sprayed inhalation, as the Chemical Corps were at a loss on how to appropriately deliver the drug, pretty much nixing any future possibility of using LSD as a large-scale weapon of war:

> Undaunted, the military surrealists and their industrial counterparts forged ahead in search of a drug and a delivery system that could do the job. During the early 1960s Edgewood Arsenal received an average of four hundred chemical "rejects" every month from the major American pharmaceutical firms. Rejects were drugs found to be commercially useless because of their undesirable side effects. Of course, undesirable side effects were precisely what the army was looking for. It was from Hoffmann-La Roche in Nutley, New Jersey, that Edgewood Arsenal obtained its first sample of a drug called quinuclidinyl benzilate, or BZ for short. The army learned that BZ inhibits the production of a chemical substance that facilitates the transfer of messages along the nerve endings, thereby disrupting normal perceptual patterns. The effects generally last about three days, although symptoms—headaches, giddiness, disorientation, auditory and visual hallucinations, and maniacal behavior—have been known to persist for as long as six weeks. "During the period of acute effects," noted an army doctor, "the person is completely out of touch with his environment." Dr. Van Sim, who served as chief of the Clinical Research Division at Edgewood, made it a practice to try all new chemicals himself before testing them on volunteers. Sim said he sampled LSD "on several occasions." Did he enjoy getting high, or were his acid trips simply a patriotic duty? "It's not a matter of compulsiveness

72

or wanting to be the first to try a material," Sim stated. "With my experience I am often able to change the design of future experiments.... This allows more comprehensive tests to be conducted later, with maximum effective usefulness of inexperienced volunteers. I'm trying to defeat the compound, and if I can, we don't have to drag out the tests at the expense of a lot of time and money." With BZ Dr. Sim seems to have met his match. "It zonked me for three days. I kept falling down and the people at the lab assigned someone to follow me around with a mattress. I woke up from it after three days without a bruise." For his efforts Sim received the Decoration for Exceptional Civilian Service and was cited for exposing himself to dangerous drugs "at the risk of grave personal injury."

According to Dr. Solomon Snyder, a leading psychopharmacologist at Johns Hopkins University, which conducted drug research for the Chemical Corps, "The army's testing of LSD was just a sideshow compared to its use of BZ." Clinical studies with EA-2277 (the code number for BZ) were initiated at Edgewood Arsenal in 1959 and continued until 1975. During this period an estimated twenty-eight hundred soldiers were exposed to the superhallucinogen. A number of military personnel have since come forward claiming that they were never the same after their encounter with BZ. Robert Bowen, a former air force enlisted man, felt disoriented for several weeks after his exposure. Bowen said the drug produced a temporary feeling of insanity but that he reacted less severely than other test subjects. One paratrooper lost all muscle control for a time and later seemed totally divorced from reality. "The last time I saw him," said Bowen, "he was taking a shower in his uniform and smoking a cigar." Pentagon spokespeople insist that the potential hazards of such experimentation were "supposed" to be fully explained to all volunteers. But as Dr. Snyder noted, nobody "can tell you for sure BZ won't have a long-lasting effect. With an initial effect of eighty hours compared to eight for LSD you would have to worry more about its long-lasting or recurrent effects." After extensive clinical testing at Edgewood Arsenal, the army concluded that BZ was better suited than LSD as a chemical warfare agent for a number of reasons. While acid could knock a person "off his rocker," to use Chemical Corps jargon, BZ would also put him "on the floor" (render him physically immobile). This unique combination—both "off the rocker" and "on the floor"—was exactly what the army sought from an incapacitant. Moreover, BZ was cheaper to produce, more reliable, and packed a stronger punch than LSD. Most important, BZ could be dispersed as an aerosol mist that would float with the wind across city or battlefield. Some advantage was also found in the fact that test subjects lapsed into a state of "semi-quiet delirium" and had no memory of their BZ experience. This was not to belittle lysergic acid. Although LSD never found a place in the army's arsenal, the drug undoubtedly left its mark on the military mind. Once again LSD seems to have acted primarily as a catalyst. Before acid touched the fancy of army strategists, Creasy's vision of a new kind of warfare was merely a pipe dream. With LSD it suddenly became a real possibility. During the early 1960s the CIA and the military began to phase out their in-house acid tests in favor of more powerful chemicals such as BZ, which became the army's standard incapacitating agent. By this time the superhallucinogen was ready for deployment in a grenade, a 750-pound cluster bomb, and at least one other largescale bomb. In addition the army tested a number of other advanced BZ munitions, including mortar, artillery, and missile warheads. The superhallucinogen was reportedly employed by American troops as a counterinsurgency weapon in Vietnam, and according to CIA documents there may be contingency plans to use the drug in the event of a major civilian insurrection. As Creasy warned shortly after he retired from the Army Chemical Corps, "We will use these things as we very well see fit, when we think it is in the best interest of the US and their allies." By the early 1960s it appeared that LSD was destined to find a niche on the pharmacologist's shelf. But then the fickle winds of medical policy began to shift. Spokesmen for the American Medical

Association (AMA) and the Food and Drug Administration started to denounce the drug, and psychedelic therapy quickly fell into public and professional disrepute. Granted, a certain amount of intransigence arises whenever a new form of treatment threatens to steal the thunder from more conventional methods, but this alone cannot account for the sudden reversal of a promising trend that was ten years in the making. One reason the medical establishment had such a difficult time coping with the psychedelic evidence was that LSD could not be evaluated like most other drugs. LSD was not a medication in the usual sense; it wasn't guaranteed to relieve a specific symptom such as a cold or headache. In this respect psychedelics were out of kilter with the basic assumptions of Western medicine. The FDA's relationship with this class of chemicals became even more problematic in light of claims that LSD could help the healthy. Most doctors automatically dismissed the notion that drugs might benefit someone who was not obviously ailing. In 1962 Congress enacted regulations that required the safety and efficacy of a new drug to be proven with respect to the condition for which it was to be marketed commercially. LSD, according to the FDA, did not satisfy these criteria. From then on, authorized distribution of the drug was tightly controlled. Anyone who wanted to work with LSD had to receive special permission from the FDA.[16]

LSD was labeled an experimental drug by the FDA, meaning it could be used for research purposes only and not as part of general psychiatric practices. Thus, it became almost impossible for psychiatrists to obtain psychedelics legally, leading some of the most distinguished and experienced investigators to abandon their work. All future works demonstrating LSD's therapeutic potential virtually vanished overnight. "It was a very intense period," recalled Dr. Oscar Janiger. "The drug experience brought together many people of diverse interests. We built up a sizeable amount of data… and then the whole thing just fell in on us. Many who formerly were regarded as groundbreakers making an important contribution suddenly found themselves disenfranchised."[17]

The psychedelic scientists were partly to blame for the FDA's bummer decision as the agency felt that too many of them had become LSD junkies. But was the FDA simply overreacting or were there other more nefarious forces at work? Up until the early 60s LSD studies had flourished without government restrictions and the CIA had sponsored a fair amount of mind control research projects. In 1962, however, LSD testing was no longer seen as a priority for the CIA, which had already learned enough about the drug to understand how it could best work in covert operations. They no longer believed that LSD could unlock the secrets of the spy trade, much less the secrets of the universe:

> While acid was still an important part of the cloak-and-dagger arsenal, by this time the CIA and the army had developed a series of superhallucinogens such as the highly touted BZ, which was thought to hold greater promise as a mind control weapon. The CIA and the military were not inhibited by the new drug laws enacted during the early 1960s. A special clause in the regulatory policy allowed the FDA to issue "selective exemptions," which meant that favored researchers would not be subject to restrictive measures. With this convenient loophole the FDA never attempted to oversee in-house pharmacological research conducted by the CIA and the military services. Secret arrangements were made whereby these organizations did not even have to file a formal "Claim for Exemption," or IND request. The FDA simply ignored all studies that were classified for reasons of national security, and CIA and military investigators were given free reign to conduct their covert experimentation. Apparently, in the eyes of the FDA, those seeking to develop hallucinogens as weapons were somehow more "sensitive to their scientific integrity and moral and ethical responsibilities" than independent researchers dedicated to exploring the therapeutic potential of LSD. In 1965 Congress passed the Drug Abuse Control Amendments, which resulted in even tighter restrictions on psychedelic research. The illicit manufacture and sale of LSD was declared a misdemeanor (oddly enough,

possession was not yet outlawed). All investigators without IND exemptions were required to turn in their remaining supplies to the FDA, which retained legal jurisdiction over psychedelics. Adverse publicity forced Sandoz to stop marketing LSD entirely in April 1966, and the number of research projects fell to a mere handful. The decision to curtail LSD experimentation was the subject of a congressional probe into the organization and coordination of federal drug research and regulatory programs. The inquiry in the spring of 1966 was led by Senator Robert Kennedy (D-NY), whose wife, Ethel, reportedly underwent LSD therapy with Dr. Ross MacLean (a close associate of Captain Hubbard's) at Hollywood Hospital in Vancouver. Senator Kennedy asked officials of the FDA and the NIMH to explain why so many LSD projects were suddenly canned. When they evaded the issue, Kennedy became annoyed. "Why if they were worthwhile six months ago, why aren't they worthwhile now?" he demanded repeatedly. The dialogue seesawed back and forth, but no satisfactory answer was forthcoming. "Why didn't you just let them continue?" asked the senator. "We keep going around and around.... If I could get a flat answer about that I would be happy. Is there a misunderstanding about my question?" Kennedy insinuated that the regulatory agencies were attempting to thwart potentially valuable research. He stressed the importance of a balanced outlook with respect to LSD: "I think we have given too much emphasis and so much attention to the fact that it can be dangerous and that it can hurt an individual who uses it... that perhaps to some extent we have lost sight of the fact that it can be very, very helpful in our society if used properly." Kennedy's plea fell on deaf ears. The FDA steadfastly refused to alter the course it had chosen. In 1967 a Psychotomimetic Advisory Committee (a joint FDA/NIMH venture) was established to process all research applications. Members of this committee included Dr. Harris Isbell and Dr. Carl Pfeiffer, two longtime CIA contract employees. Shortly thereafter the NIMH terminated its last in-house LSD project involving human subjects. In

1968 the Drug Abuse Control Amendments were modified to make possession of LSD a misdemeanor and sale a felony. Responsibility for enforcing the law was shifted from the FDA to the newly formed Bureau of Narcotics and Dangerous Drugs. Two years later psychedelic drugs were placed in the Schedule I category—a classification reserved for drugs of abuse that have no medical value.[18]

Around the same time that the government began to eliminate LSD it was too late; as word of the drug began to spread, access to psychedelic therapists became harder to find. Yet, an eager populace wouldn't be denied, finding new avenues to catch the rainbow. A psychedelic-fueled curiosity had gained momentum with the public, and quickly reached a point where the government could no longer contain it. The CIA now had a black market acid extravaganza they helped to create, but now had to control, as LSD hit the streets as acid blotter sheets to meet the growing demand. The rise of this remarkable social phenomenon continued to gather strength despite the admonitions of educators, doctors, politicians and the CIA's mad scientists that created a new generation of Frankensteins—embellished in their own laboratories that stretched across America—as millions of young explorers conducted their own experiments with LSD.

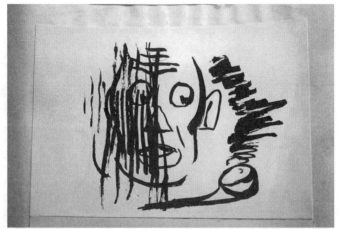

A drawing made by one of the participant in the Bulgarian LSD tests
(*Atlas Obscura*)

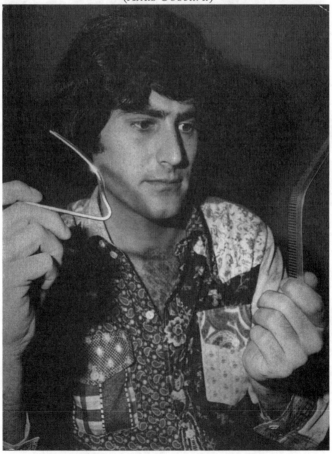

Uri Geller (*Hulton Archive / Getty Images*)

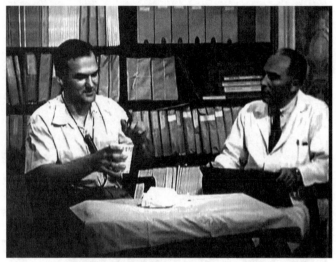

William Millarc takes LSD in 1955,
while Dr. Bercel interviews him on film

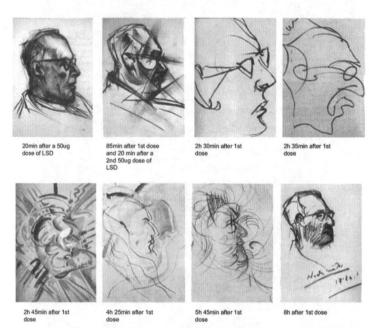

20min after a 50ug
dose of LSD

85min after 1st dose
and 20 min after a
2nd 50ug dose of
LSD

2h 30min after 1st
dose

2h 35min after 1st
dose

2h 45min after 1st
dose

4h 25min after 1st
dose

5h 45min after 1st
dose

8h after 1st dose

Drawings made by an artist under the influence of LSD

Chapter Four

Timothy Leary, Harvard
and the LSD Beatniks

*I was halfway across America, at the dividing line between
the East of my youth and the West of my future.*
—Jack Kerouac, *On the Road*

"Anyone who wanted to take the voyage is welcome to come along," Timothy Leary told a group of students at Harvard, enticing them to join him for a psychedelic session outside the university. Leary, a Harvard psychologist turned acid evangelist was tall, good looking, with a full head of wavy gray-peppered hair and a bright smile—the future godfather of LSD had charisma for days. It's no wonder that the man who turned America on was watched closely by the CIA for decades. But before Leary turned on, tuned in and dropped out he was just another "anonymous institutional employee who drove to work each morning in a long line of commuter cars and drove home each night and drank martinis... like several million middle-class, liberal, intellectual robots"[1] despite the perceived success of being a Harvard doctor. In a matter of years he would be on a quest to turn on as many as people as possible to LSD and no spooks, cops, or corrupt government agencies were going to stop him.

Harvard graduate students and selected beatnik artists like Allen Ginsberg flocked to his unlikely suburban home on Homer Street in Newton, a suburb of Cambridge where the university was located. The magnificent home, a lavender three-story Georgian Revival was built by a wealthy bicycle manufacturer in the 1890s, with leaded-glass windows, and fleur-de-lis tiles inside the fireplace. Its walls would soon be turned to graffitied art slogans while the floorboards of its porch became charred from ill-advised bonfires. Such was the setting for many a good trip. Beatnik poet Allen Ginsberg arrived with his lover Peter Orlovsky at Leary's house in Newton just in time for Christmas in 1960. Ginsberg had taken LSD the previous year at a research institute in Palo Alto, California but this would be his first experience with psilocybin, which was currently on the menu at Leary's house.

The Harvard doctor had his first bite of magic mushrooms in the hills of Oaxaca, Mexico after being persuaded by a *Life* magazine article and a friendly executive from JP Morgan. The psychologist traveled to Cuernavaca, Mexico and purchased some mushrooms from a local curandera but skipped the colorfully loud shroom eating ritual, instead choosing to eat them by the pool of his villa. It had an instant impact on the forty-year old doctor. "I learned more about my brain and its possibilities and more about psychology in the five hours after taking these mushrooms than in the preceding 15 years of studying and doing research in psychology,"[2] he later recalled.

Leary returned to Harvard and sought out fresh doses of psilocybin, and he acquired a fresh batch from—where else— Sandoz, of course. With his partner and colleague Dr. Richard Alpert (the future Ram Dass) and Aldous Huxley on board, Leary formed the Harvard Psilocybin Project. He had many patients, including the two poets Ginsberg and Orlovsky, a gay couple who were under Leary's guidance after swallowing the magic mushroom pills. Soon, to the dismay of their host, the lovers would be naked and swimming around on the living room floor with supernatural beams in their eyes. Ginsberg even telephoned beatnik godfather Jack Kerouac, author of *On the Road*, the bible of the beat generation; although Kerouac only lived a half hour away he was caring for his mother and declined to come to trip with them over at Leary's house. Eventually the high wore off and it left Ginsberg with a feeling that his experience held implications far beyond the known world of medicine and psychology. He began to ask questions of Leary who in response suggested that if psychedelic drugs held the promise of changing mankind and ushering in a new era of humanity, then they would have to be available to the average citizen and not just doctors and spooks. Leary was one of the unsuspecting doctors entrusted by the CIA to study psychedelic drugs. One couldn't ask for a much more prestigious university to work at than Harvard; it was after the all the alma mater of then president John F. Kennedy. The agency could have never predicted that Leary, a respected academic and serious scientist with short hair and nerdy getup, would go on to lead the chemical revolution. Perhaps things might have turned out much differently if Ginsberg didn't fill up his head with thoughts about love and peace in a psychedelic utopia. The poet later noted, "that the very technology stereotyping our consciousness and desensitizing our perceptions should throw up its own antidote... Given such historic Comedy, who should emerge from Harvard University but the one and only Dr. Leary, a respectable human being, a worldly man faced with the task of a Messiah."[3] And messiah he became while spearheading a movement looking to transform human consciousness with the power of psychedelics. Leary proclaimed, "We were thinking far-out history thoughts at Harvard, believing that it was time (after the shallow and nostalgic fifties) for far-out visions, knowing that America had run out of philosophy, that a new empirical, tangible metaphysics was desperately needed; knowing in our hearts that the old mechanical myths had died at Hiroshima, that the past was over, and that politics could not fill the spiritual vacuum."[4]

Leary believed that by changing the drugs you could change your heart, and since the drugs of the time were alcohol, coffee and cigarettes it was time to ditch those and get with the far more healthy and spiritual option—psychedelics: "Politics, religion, economics, social structure, are based on shared states of consciousness. The cause of social conflict is usually neurological. The cure is biochemical."[5]

It was a formidable task but Leary, Ginsberg and others of generation beat were up to it. Soon Ginsberg was combing through his little black book and marking down the names of people they could turn on. Ginsberg was the most important poet of his time and a cultural ambassador of the arts; he jetted back to New York with a stash of psilocybin pills, recruiting soldiers for his chemical army:

> At the Five Spot in Greenwich Village he gave the mushroom pills to Theolonius Monk, the great jazz pianist. A few days later Ginsberg dropped by Monk's apartment to check on the results. Monk peered out from behind a crack in the door, smiled, and asked if he had anything stronger.

Ginsberg also turned on Dizzy Gillespie, who was evidently quite pleased by the gesture. "Oh yeah," he laughed, "anything that gets you high." In a sense it was Ginsberg's way of returning a historical favor; the jazz musicians had given marijuana to the beats, and now the beats were turning the jazz cats on to psychedelics. Word of the new drugs spread quickly through the jazz scene, and numerous musicians, including many of the preeminent players in the field experimented with psychedelics in the early 1960s. John Coltrane, the acknowledged master of the tenor saxophone, took LSD and reported upon returning from his inner voyage that he "perceived the interrelationship of all life forms." It was through Ginsberg that the existence of Leary's research project came to the attention of the beat network…Another writer Ginsberg brought into Leary's circle was the poet Charles Olson, formerly rector of Black Mountain College in North Carolina. A man of overpowering intellect, Olson was fifty years old at the time of his psychedelic initiation. He stood a towering six feet seven inches, had unruly strands of white hair, and spoke in a deep resonant voice. Olson remembered the first time he tried psilocybin: "I was so high on bourbon that I took it as though it was a bunch of peanuts. I kept throwing the peanuts—and the mushroom into my mouth." He described the experience as [a] "love feast, a truth pill… it makes you exactly what you are." Olson had a strong affinity for the mushroom. He thought it a "wretched shame that we don't have it in the common drugstore as a kind of beer, because it's so obviously an attractive and useful, normal food." But he also sensed immediately that psychedelics were a profound threat to the status quo. After the drug wore off, his first words to Leary were, "When they come after you, you can hide at my house." Leary, being an apolitical creature, shrugged off the remark without much thought. Little did he know that the CIA was already keeping an eye on his escapades at Harvard.[6]

But Leary had chutzpah and his chemical quest continued as he sought out William Burroughs, the famed author of *Naked*

Lunch, a somewhat mentor of the beat generation. Burroughs had a legendary curiosity and most certainly would try anything once. By the time Leary arrived in Tangiers, where the writer was living in the summer of 1961, he was smoking copious amounts of Moroccan hash and experimenting with a hallucination causing flicker machine. But his psilocybin trip with Leary was a bummer that went from a moonlight swim to spending time in seclusion. Despite this he agreed to join Leary back at Harvard for more psychedelic tests and further experiments in altered states of consciousness. Things like sensory deprivation tanks and other far-out technical wonders that a prestigious university should have interested the shit out of Burroughs, but upon arriving in Cambridge all he kept hearing about was some intellectual jive about cosmic brotherly love. Leary kept touting the psilocybin pills as a form of enlightenment therapy, a needed cure-all for a rapidly declining world, but Burroughs was a mind-expanding veteran who lectured Leary about the darker side of American politics. Despite their high hopes for hallucinogens Burroughs cautioned that sinister forces were most likely also interested in these drugs and probably not for the same reasons. Burroughs left Leary by warning him that they might be playing right into their hands. The iconic writer feared that the government would use psychedelics to control the zombie masses rather than to liberate them. He was basically right, but it wouldn't be psychedelics that turned the masses of the future into zombies. Burroughs basically dissed Leary and the rest of the beat generation hoping for a chemical revolution in the opening passages of *Nova Express*, published in 1964:

> At the immediate risk of finding myself the most unpopular character of all fiction—and history is fiction—I must say this: "Bring together state of news—Inquire onward from state to doer—Who monopolized Immortality? Who monopolized Cosmic Consciousness? Who monopolized Love Sex and Dream? Who monopolized Life Time and Fortune? Who took from you what is yours? Now they will give it all back? Did they ever give anything away for nothing? Did they ever give any more than they had to give? Did they not always take back what they gave when possible

and it always was? Listen: Their Garden Of Delights is a terminal sewer—I have been at some pains to map this area of terminal sewage in the so called pornographic sections of *Naked Lunch* and *Soft Machine*—Their Immortality Cosmic Consciousness and Love is second-run grade-B shit—Their drugs are poison designed to beam in Orgasm Death and Nova Ovens—Stay out of the Garden Of Delight—It is a man-eating trap that ends in green goo—Throw back their ersatz Immortality—It will fall apart before you can get out of The Big Store—flush their drug kicks down the drain— They are poisoning and monopolizing the hallucinogen drugs—learn to make it without any chemical corn—All that they offer is a screen to cover retreat from the colony they have so disgracefully managed. To cover travel arrangements so they will never have to pay the constituents they have betrayed and sold out. Once these arrangements are complete they will blow the place up behind them. And what does my program of total austerity and total resistance offer you? I offer you nothing. I am not a politician. These are conditions of total emergency. And these are my instructions for total emergency if carried out now could avert the total disaster now on tracks: "Peoples of the earth, you have all been poisoned... I order total resistance directed against this conspiracy to pay off peoples of the earth in ersatz bullshit."[7]

With Burroughs out of the picture Leary was a bit disappointed but he carried on pushing the magic mushroom pills until a figure arrived on the scene that had such a huge impact on him that it literally changed the course of history. This figure of destiny was Michael Hollingshead, an artful Englishman that came across a full gram of LSD-25 while living in New York City. After mixing the LSD with powdered sugar and distilled water, it was spooned into a mayonnaise jar and stored away for future trips. Hollingshead's first trip was so mind blowing that he called Aldous Huxley and asked him what to do next as Hollingshead was confused whether LSD was illuminating or dangerous. One hit of the drug had destroyed his sense of self as he later noted: "The reality on which I had consciously based my personality had dissolved into maya, a hallucinatory facade. Stripped of one kind of reality, and unwilling or unable to benefit from the possibilities of another one, I was acutely aware of my helplessness, my utter transience, my suspension between two worlds, one outside and the other wholly within."[8]

Besides suffering a psychedelic-revealed inward crises, Hollingshead was also financially broken and suffering marital problems. Seeing what seemed like a future destined for a spot on the shrink's couch, Huxley suggested that he head to Harvard to meet Timothy Leary, because If there was any mental investigator worth seeing, it was him. Hollingshead obliged and drove off for Cambridge with his magic mayonnaise jar. Leary greeted the Englishman with hospitality and offered him a free room in his attic, gave him some walking around money and invited Hollingshead to join the psilocybin research team. Hollingshead enjoyed the psilocybin session, but confided to Leary that the drug wasn't nearly as strong as LSD. Leary laughed, believing that all psychedelics were the same and even though Hollingshead offered his host some, Leary declined. He was the one studying the effects of psychedelia and not the other way around. Hollingshead shrugged and went on with his business. A few nights later he was driving around outside Leary's house with the funky trumpeter Maynard Ferguson and his wife, smoking a joint inside the car while trying to convince them to try a taste of his magic mayonnaise. After killing the joint they went inside the house where Hollingshead zoomed up the stairs to fetch his mayonnaise jar. All three took a hit and within an hour the LSD was starting to kick their asses. When Leary walked into the living room and saw the looks on their faces, glowing like electric toasters, he wanted to know more. Did he dare join in? Hollingshead took a heaping spoonful, and offered it up to the Harvard Doctor. Leary hesitated but relented, downing the glob of sugary LSD in one swift swallow. Soon he was flying as he later recalled in *High Priest*:

> It took about a half-hour to hit. And it came sudden and irresistible. An endless deep swamp marsh of some other planet teeming and steaming with energy and life, and in the swamp an enormous tree whose branches were foliated out miles high and miles wide. And then this tree,

like a cosmic vacuum cleaner, went ssssuuuck, and every cell in my body was swept into the root, twigs, branches, and leaves of this tree. Tumbling and spinning, down the soft fibrous avenues to some central point which was just light. Just light, but not just light. It was the center of Life. A burning, dazzling, throbbing, radiant core, pure pulsing, exulting light. A endless flame that contained everything— sound, touch, cell, seed, sense, soul, sleep, glory, glorifying, God, the hard eye of God. Merged with this pulsing flame it was possible to look out and see and participate in the entire cosmic drama. Past and future. All forms, all structures, all organisms, all events, were illusory, television productions pulsing out from the central eye.[9]

The power of LSD shook Leary to his core as he wandered around the house dazed and confused, contemplating questions he never dreamed to ask before. Questions about his strict Catholic upbringing as an only child abandoned by his father. Questions about the mother of his children who committed suicide while Leary was sleeping, leaving him to fend for himself in caring for their two kids. For days Leary was a mess as he latched onto the Englishman Hollingshead like he was some sort of guru, following him around, asking the strangest of questions, convinced that the pot-bellied prankster was a cosmic messenger.

His colleagues thought that Leary had finally blown his mind until Hollingshead gave every member of the psilocybin project a hit of LSD, samples of which blew their minds as well. From that moment on LSD became the king of the campus as an air of mystery and excitement started to float over the hallowed halls of Harvard. With his jar of magic mayonnaise Hollingshead had turned on the legendary institute of higher learning. He later warned, "LSD involved risk. It was anarchistic; it upset our applecarts, torpedoed our cherished illusions, sabotaged our beliefs... Yet there were some of my circle who, with Rimbaud, could say, 'I dreamed of crusades, senseless voyages of discovery, republics without a history, moral revolution, displacement of races and continents. I believed in all the magics.'"[10]

After turning on Leary. Hollingshead went back to London in

September 1965, strapped with enough LSD to produce 5,000 trips, along with thirteen boxes of psychedelic literature and plans for a psychedelic jam at the Royal Albert Hall with the Beatles and the Stones. Intent on bringing the psychedelic revolution to England, Hollingshead set up shop at his flat in Belgravia's Pont Street, which he renamed the World Psychedelic Centre. Hollingshead's Centre was one of only two reliable sources for LSD in London at the time, and was a natural pilgrimage for artists wanting to turn on including Roman Polanski, Alex Trocchi, Eric Clapton, Donovan and the Rolling Stones—all of whom stopped by to partake in LSD sessions decorated with comfy cushions, the latest stereo hi-fi equipment, a movie projector and other provisions needed for a good trip. The LSD was usually dispensed after midnight with grapes infused with 300 micrograms of the drug. A chill atmosphere was key, and music helped. Hollingshead writes:

> Shortly after dropping the acid, I played a tape of Buddhist Chakra music, followed by Concert Percussion by the American composer, John Cage. Next I played some music by Ravi Shankar and some bossanova. Interval of fifteen minutes. Then some music by Scriabin and part of a Bach cello suite. Interval. Some Debussy, and Indian flute music by Ghosh. Interval. Bach organ music and some John Cage 'space' music. Interval. The Ali Brothers and Japanese flute music. We also looked at slides projected on to the ceiling of Tantric yantras, Vedic Gods, the Buddha, Tibetan mandalas. There were also regular readings from Leary's work.[11]

While Hollingshead dispensed LSD to his visitors in carefully controlled conditions, in a similar way that Leary would do after leaving Harvard, he was soon seen in the tabloids as an evil criminal dispersing killer drugs to the British youth. After hosting an LSD party where two undercover police officers were dosed after sampling the spiked punch, Hollingshead was busted and sentenced to two years at Wormwood Scrubs, a Victorian-era prison in Hammersmith. Hollingshead smuggled in some LSD and turned on the KGB spy George Blake before making a break for it, escaping to

Cumbrae, a Scottish island, where he settled with a group of people that he soon turned into believers. Hollingshead, now an exile and escaped fugitive traveled the world from Norway to Nepal before writing the semi-autobiographical *The Man Who Turned on the World*, published in 1973. Undoubtedly a key player in the LSD scene, Hollingshead's influence in the psychedelic revolution would soon be forgotten as his addiction to opiates, alcohol and speed led him to a mysterious death in Bolivia. But back in the early days of LSD, Hollingshead provided plenty of Psychedelic magic to would-be seekers of a new age of enlightenment.

But the magic was wearing thin, at least according to a confidential memorandum issued by the CIA's Office of Security, suggesting that certain agents were involved with Leary's group at Harvard. They wanted to make sure that these hallucinogenic drugs could be controlled and if they weren't able to do so, then they wanted them branded as extremely dangerous. The once classified document concluded clearly that:

> Information concerning the use of this type of drug for experimental or personal reasons should be reported immediately...In addition, any information of Agency personnel involved with Drs. ALPERT or LEARY, or with any other group engaged in this type of activity should also be reported.[12]

During this period Leary was handing out LSD to almost everyone, including Mary Pinchot, an artist and prominent socialite who was married to high-ranking CIA goon Cord Meyer. Leary and Pinchot struck up a friendship without him ever knowing who her husband worked for, and soon he was teaching her how to give guided trips and plying her with doses of the drug to distribute to her wealthy friends back in Georgetown. Pinchot later told Leary, "I can't give you all the details, but top people in Washington are turning on. You'd be amazed at the sophistication of some of our leaders. We're getting a little group together..."[13] Leary didn't know that Mary Pinchot was one of many girlfriends that President Kennedy was banging during his time as president. The two smoked weed together in the White House a few times, and it's likely that

Pinchot infamously dosed JFK with her LSD-filled eyedropper. Less than a year later, Kennedy would be dead and shortly after so would Pinchot, both murdered by rogue elements within the CIA. When Leary learned of her death, all of their conversations about LSD came back to him, including the times she hinted that the CIA was watching him. Leary recalled how Pinchot warned him that if his research stuck solely with magic mushrooms the company would leave him alone, but if he continued to let his LSD experiments get out of hand, he might find himself put out of business.

Soon CIA MK-ULTRA mind control veterans like Dr. Max Rinkel and Dr. Robert Heath were denouncing Leary in the Harvard Alumni Review and by 1962, the Boston press. This prompted an investigation by the US Food and Drug Administration that promptly shut down his psychedelic operation. Leary and associates grudgingly surrendered their supplies of psilocybin and LSD to the university. Leary believed that the establishment had a plan to keep psychedelics out of the hands of everyday Joes, and accused the government and the medical industrial complex of conspiring to suppress valuable psychedelic research. Leary later acquired some LSD from superspy Captain Al Hubbard, the other acid pioneer who also warned him about pissing off the CIA. "I liked Tim when we first met, but I warned him a dozen times… I gave stuff to Leary and he turned out to be completely no good… He seemed like a well-intentioned person, but then he went overboard."[14] Leary's approach to research methodology included sugar cubes laced with LSD that had half the students on the Harvard campus tripping balls. When his superiors had finally had enough and fired him, Leary remarked, "LSD is so powerful, that one administered dose can start a thousand rumors." For Leary and his outfit of psychedelic vagabonds it was just the beginning of a long strange trip that nobody, except for maybe the CIA saw coming:

> In May 1963 Richard Alpert was summarily dismissed from his teaching post for violating an agreement not to give LSD to undergraduate students. It was the first time a Harvard faculty member had been fired in the twentieth century. "Some day it will be quite humorous," he told a reporter, "that a professor was fired for supplying a student with 'the most

profound educational experience in my life.' That's what he told the Dean it was." A few days later the academic axe fell on Leary as well, after he failed to attend an honors program committee meeting—a rather paltry excuse, but by this time the university higher-ups were glad to get rid of him on any pretext. Leary was unruffled by the turn of events. LSD, he stated tersely, was "more important than Harvard." He and Alpert fired off a declaration to the Harvard Review blasting the university as "the Establishment's apparatus for training consciousness contractors," an "intellectual ministry of defense." The Harvard scandal was hot news. In the coming months most of the major US magazines featured stories on LSD and its foremost proponent. Leary was suddenly "Mr. LSD," and he welcomed the publicity. The extensive media coverage doubtless spurred the growth of the psychedelic underground. Rebuffed by the academic and medical authorities, Leary decided to take his case directly to the people—in particular, young people. He was convinced that the revelation and revolution were at hand. The hope for the future rested on a simple equation: the more who turned on, the better.[15]

Leary morphed into the High Priest of acid, urging people to "Turn on, tune in, and drop out," and as the media helped spread his gospel throughout the land the CIA watched in the shadows licking their lips in stoned disbelief. Leary had unwittingly fanned the flames of a social experiment the agency was trying to contain. Soon they would all become unwilling agents of a drug far too powerful to control or understand, as a band of west coast merry pranksters began spreading LSD to the common folks in the most infamous psychedelic road trip of all times. As a new decade dawned the cat was finally out of the bag and it wasn't munching on catnip.

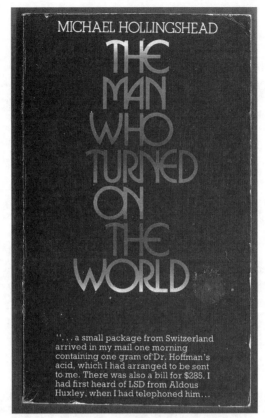

The Man Who Turned on the World (*Pinterest*)

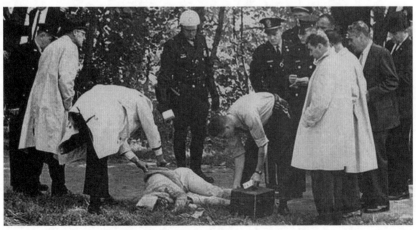

Mary Pinchot's Murder Scene (*AP*)

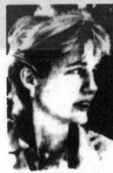

Woman Artist Shot To Death On Stroll In Washington

Robbery Believed Motive; Suspect Caught, Identified

WASHINGTON, Oct. 13 (AP)
Georgetown artist Mary Pinchot Meyer was shot to death yesterday afternoon as she walked along the path of an old canal where she often had strolled with Mrs. John F. Kennedy.

Mrs Meyer, who would have been 44 tomorrow, was a niece of Gifford Pinchot, progressive conservationist and two-term governor of Pennsylvania, and the daughter of Amos Pinchot, a found-

—Associated Press Wirephoto
MARY PINCHOT MEYER
Niece of governor

a writer employed by the Central Intelligence Agency. He was one of the founders of the United World Federalists, Inc., and a memebr of the U S. delegation to the United Nations conference in San Francisco in 1945.

An abstract painter, Mrs. Meyer has exhibited work in several Washington galleries. A collection of her paintings currently is on tour of Latin America under the auspices of the Pan American Union. The Meyers had two sons, Quentin, 18, who attends the Salisbury School in Salisbury Conn., and Mark, 14, a student at the Milton Academy near Boston.

Saw Struggle

Henry Wiggins, 24, told police he was driving his tow truck along the canal when he heard a scream and saw a woman struggling with a man. As Mr. Wiggins got out of his truck he heard two shots. When he reached the retainer

Newspaper Clipping of Pinchot's Death

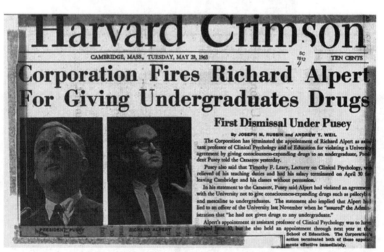

Harvard Crimson

CAMBRIDGE, MASS., TUESDAY, MAY 28, 1963   TEN CENTS

Corporation Fires Richard Alpert For Giving Undergraduates Drugs

First Dismissal Under Pusey

By JOSEPH M. RUSSIN and ANDREW T. WEIL

The Corporation has terminated the appointment of Richard Alpert as assistant professor of Clinical Psychology and of Education for violating a University agreement by giving consciousness-expanding drugs to an undergraduate, President Pusey told the Crimson yesterday.

Pusey also said that Timothy F. Leary, Lecturer on Clinical Psychology, was relieved of his teaching duties and had his salary terminated on April 30 for leaving Cambridge and his classes without permission.

In his statement to the Crimson, Pusey said Alpert had violated an agreement with the University not to give consciousness-expanding drugs such as psilocybin and mescaline to undergraduates. The statement also implied that Alpert had lied to an officer of the University last November when he "assured" the Administration that "he had not given drugs to any undergraduate."

Alpert's appointment as assistant professor of Clinical Psychology was to have ended June 30, but he also held an appointment through next year at the School of Education. The Corporation's action terminated both of these appointments effective immediately.

PRESIDENT PUSEY   RICHARD ALPERT

Newspaper Clipping announcing the firing of Dr. Richard Alpert
(*Harvard Crimson*)

Chapter Five

Taste the Electric Kool Aid:
Ken Kesey's Magic Bus Ride

*I always thought that this is one of those things that
proves God has a sense of humor. Once I realized that it
was the CIA that turned on America.*
—Ken Kesey

While the CIA was starting to worry that Leary's freewheeling LSD trips were getting out of hand and looked to put a lid on it, they had no idea that a far bigger monster was about to hatch out west. They had already been sponsoring secret LSD tests around the country, most of them in outdated veteran's and mental hospitals. The patients, mostly unwitting kooks, junkies or shopworn veterans were easily disposable staples of society. It's in this environment at the Menlo Park Veteran's hospital that a starving college student named Ken Kesey would be exposed to LSD for the first time as he signed up for the test eager for the $25 bucks they were offering. At that time Kesey was your typical straight-laced student bumming his way as an undergrad at Stanford University's creative writing program in 1960.

Originally from Oregon, Kesey didn't smoke or drink alcohol and never had any experiences with drugs of any sort. He might have been the soberest man in all of California. He wouldn't be for long. Like Ginsberg and so many before him, Kesey was about to embark on a CIA-sponsored psychedelic trip as a human guinea pig in the study of psychotomimetic drugs. Kesey, a blue-eyed lumberjack and former high school wrestling champion, downed the LSD and blasted off into the universe as a neon phoenix, returning in metaphysical ashes a whole new man after plummeting back to earth, or California—wherever the fuck he was. By the trip's third hour he was intrigued by the mechanics of the microphone taping his speech as he contemplated the vastness of the universe while staring through the checkered metal windows. All the nurses looked like frogmen, and by the time he had come down, Kesey was so blown away by the experience that he asked for a job at the hospital. A few weeks later he was working the janitorial night shift in the psychiatric ward, where he had access to a plethora of psychedelic goodies like LSD, mescaline, Ditran, and the mysterious IT-290 (Alpha-Methyltryptamine). At first Kesey sparingly pillaged these drugs which he circulated among friends in Stanford's bohemian village of Perry Lane.

When he wasn't writing or going to school he was working as a janitor at the hospital, tripping on LSD and pondering the limits of insanity while pushing a mop. Kesey recalled, "Before I took drugs, I didn't know why the guys in the psycho ward at the VA Hospital were there. I didn't understand them. After I took LSD, suddenly I saw it. I saw it all. I listened to them and watched them, and I saw that what they were saying and doing was not so crazy after all."[1] Kesey's first novel, *One Flew Over the Cuckoo's Nest*, was starting to percolate out of him, inspired by his time tripping and working at Menlo Park. Soon Kesey had turned on almost the entire Perry Lane community, as a psychedelic party scene began to emerge. Eventually Kesey stole all the psychedelic drugs at the hospital and never looked back as he went on to start the famous acid tests in the San Francisco Bay area, and was really the godfather of the West

coast acid movement. All thanks to the CIA, who basically provided the seemingly endless supply of the drugs failing, to foresee the impact they'd have once unleashed on society. With bowls full of LSD-spiked chili, Kesey dined electric with artists like Roy Sebum, writers such as Larry McMurtry and a young unknown musician named Jerry Garcia. The tripping college kids developed a taste for psychedelics and even ordered a box of peyote buttons from a company in Texas back when it was still legal.

Peyote, a powerful Native American sacrament, was known for producing spirit visions and after ingesting a few buttons, Kesey had a vision of a strong Indian Chief. This vision propelled him to create Chief Broom, a schizophrenic Indian, as the main character in the novel he was writing at the time—*One Flew Over the Cuckoo's Nest*. Almost the entire book was written while Kesey was either tripping on LSD or peyote buttons. When released, the book received fabulous reviews and was both a critical and commercial success, much to the surprise of Kesey who was now viewed in the eyes of the establishment as the most interesting and prominent character of the emerging psychedelic scene. Kesey, just a short while earlier working as a janitor, was now all of a sudden a literary whirlwind with a chance at writing the Great American Novel. With his royalties he bought a country home in La Honda, and began work on his second novel, his love letter to Oregon and magnum opus *Some Great Notion*. His country house in La Honda soon became a retreat for beatniks, intellectuals, artists and acidheads who all swayed to the rock music blasting out of Kesey's mammoth outdoor speakers that welcomed visitors as they hung over the porch. About an hour south of San Francisco, the antics at Kesey's home saw the birth of the Merry Pranksters, a group of fun-loving acid enthusiasts bound for the most epic road trip ever:

> The Pranksters purchased a 1939 International Harvester school bus and refurbished it with bunks, refrigerators, shelves, and a sink. They put a hole in the roof so people could sit up top and play music, and they wired the entire vehicle so they could broadcast from within and pick up sounds from outside as well. En masse the Pranksters swarmed over the weather-beaten body with paintbrushes, producing the first psychedelic motor transport done in bright, swirling colors. A sign hung on the rear end which read, "Caution: Weird Load." Emblazoned on the front of the bus was the word "FURTHUR" (with two u's), which aptly summed up the Prankster ethos. There were twenty-odd people aboard, and the entire crew was ready for "the great freak forward." The Pranksters dressed in elaborate costumes, donning capes and masks, painting themselves with Day-Glo, and wearing pieces of the American flag. They took names befitting their new psychedelic identities.

Among the women were Mountain Girl, Sensuous X, Gretchen Fetchin the Slime Queen, and Doris Delay. Ken Babbs was Intrepid Traveler. The magnetic Kesey was Swashbuckler. And Mike Hagen, trying to keep his movie camera steady while the bus lurched down the road, was Mal Function. The Pranksters were constantly filming an epic saga that would star everybody. Kesey's slogan—"Get them into your movie before they get you into theirs"—was not just a conviction but a strategy. As they disembarked from the bus with the loudspeakers blasting rock and roll, the Pranksters were well aware that they looked to straight citizens like inhabitants of another planet. That was exactly what they intended. They were into "tootling the multitudes," doing whatever was necessary to blow minds and keep folks off balance. "The purpose of psychedelics," said Kesey, "is to learn the conditioned responses of people and then to prank them. That's the only way to get people to ask questions, and until they ask questions they're going to remain conditioned robots."[2]

The pranksters rolled into Phoenix during the 1964 presidential campaign decked out in American flag regalia in support of ultra-conservative Barry Goldwater. Driving the technicolor bus was Neal Cassady, the aging avatar beatnik fresh from a two-year stint in San Quentin for possessing one joint of marijuana. He was now a speed freak, trimmed and cut by a brutal prison sentence, yet still jovial and commanding—when he wasn't shoving his face full of amphetamines. It's no wonder why Cassady was the driver, being much like the truckers before and after him that relied on speed to get through long stretches of driving. The Pranksters were greeted with curiosity and enthusiasm as they retraced the mythic roads traversed by the beat protagonists years before, although this time it wasn't conga grooves and poetry they were dishing out—it was acid. The Pranksters doled the drug out like candy to any and all during their road trip; they themselves drank from an electric jug of orange juice where nobody knew the dosage, but everyone knew the trip. By the time the CIA caught wind of what was going on, the Pranksters were zigzagging stoned immaculate through the Blue Ridge Mountains, defying death as they rode towards the Big Apple after Johnny Apple-seeding the country with LSD in an attempt to wake up the nation. When the Pranksters finally hit New York City or what they called "Madhattan" they were in high spirits, eager to explore the village and turn on the stuffy socialites of 5th Avenue. Upon arrival, Kesey phoned his agent, Sterling Lord, and a powwow was setup between the old and new godfathers of the beat generation. Lord remembered:

Although Cassady was friends with Kesey and Kerouac, the two writers met only once, and that was while the Pranksters were in New York on this trip. Kesey and the Pranksters were staying in a vacant Manhattan apartment owned by a cousin of one member of the group. The apartment was in a building on Madison Avenue between 89th and 90th streets. Further was parked in front of the 90th Street Pharmacy on the other side of Madison Avenue for about a week. Ken and several other Pranksters were eager to meet Jack because they had been deeply influenced by *On the Road*. I told Kerouac that Kesey was going to be in town and would be in touch with him. Cassady contacted Allen Ginsberg, and the two of them, along with Peter Orlovsky, Allen's partner, and Peter's brother Julius, who was one day out of a 14-year stay in a mental institution, drove out to Northport on Long Island to pick up Kerouac and bring him into Manhattan. Jack was 12 years older than Ken, and there was a marked difference in their energies and interests. Jack had been living in a house with his mother in Northport, although he still had to deal from time to time with the public adulation inspired by the 1957 publication of *On the Road*. His was a relatively passive life. Kesey and the Pranksters, on the other hand, were on an extended high that peaked in New York. According to one of the Pranksters, Ken Babbs, every place they had stopped on the bus trip, they had gotten out their musical instruments, donned their regalia, turned on the cameras and tape recorders, and broken into "spontaneous combustion musical and verbal make-believe shenanigans." The Pranksters were still doing a version of this in the New York City apartment. This was the atmosphere into which Kerouac walked. Unlike the intrepid Pranksters, Jack sat quietly on the side, "slightly aloof," as Babbs told me. They draped a small American flag over Jack's shoulders, but he took it off, folded it neatly, and placed it on the arm of the couch. There was absolutely no serious or colorful discussion between Kesey and Kerouac. Jack was never loud, or critical, or indignant. He seemed tired, but he was patient with the Pranksters' antics. Still, an hour after he came, he left. In the end, he was uncomfortable with Kesey's overwhelming display of exuberance. But the Kerouac-Kesey encounter carried a message: Ken Kesey was not a part of the Beat Generation. Thanks to a CIA-funded drug experiment at a veterans hospital, which had introduced Kesey to psychedelic drugs, Kesey instead sparked the Psychedelic Revolution, which spawned the hippie movement. Kesey brought LSD to people's awareness, and he and the Merry Pranksters spoke of its mind-expanding, life-enhancing properties... The Beats and the Pranksters showed us different ways of opting out of society. They were both countercultural movements. The Beats were trying to change literature, and the Pranksters were trying to change the people and the country.[3]

Kesey's meeting with Kerouac was a dud but the upbeat, freedom-loving spirit of the Pranksters was still alive. As the once relevant writer Kerouac left the party, Tom Wolfe, the scribe of the expedition later described the meeting of the cross-generational writers; "It was like hail and farewell. Kerouac was the old star. Kesey was the wild new comet from the West heading christ knew where."[4] Wolfe's account of the magic bus ride that changed America, *The Electric Kool Aid Acid Test,* was a massive best-seller that made Kesey more famous as a cultural curiosity than he ever was as a writer. And while his meeting with Kerouac was a bummer, he had high hopes for Timothy Leary's group, now settled in Millbrook, a psychedelic commune in upstate New

York. Besides their own acid enclaves in the Bay area, Leary's compound was the only other LSD retreat they knew of, and after driving thousands of miles they sure couldn't pass up on the opportunity to trip with Leary, the legendary doctor of East Coast LSD.

But first they went to the World's Fair which they found not to be a very cool place at all, despite all the promises of a future wonderland. It turned out the Fair got their world of tomorrow all wrong; the future wasn't a white utopia with space age furniture, but a multi-colored acid trip with guitar riffs from Mars. Furthur the bus rolled into Leary's compound, a 4,000 acre spread, thick with trees, wildlife and the sounds of distant waterfalls. The quiet serene setting was interrupted with smoke bombs, trumpet flares and the overall noisy grand arrival of Kesey's Merry Pranksters. Most people at the house vanished except for Ram Dass who greeted the Pranksters alone. The Pranksters, expecting to be greeted with open arms, were somewhat miffed that upon their arrival to the sprawling mansion, they weren't exactly embraced. Also, that momentous meeting between Kesey and Leary never materialized, as the doctor refused to come downstairs to meet them. Supposedly Leary was in the midst of a serious three-day trip and couldn't be disturbed:

> Kesey was bewildered by this turn of events, but as the Pranksters grew more familiar with the Millbrook scene, they began to understand why they made everyone so uptight. The Millbrook group was essentially made up of behavioral scientists who kept records of their mental states, wrote papers, and put out a journal. Leary and his people were going the scholarly route, giving lectures and such; they had nothing to gain by associating with a bunch of grinning, filthy bums wearing buckskins and face paint. The distance between the East Coast intellectuals and Kesey's clan was cavernous. As Michael Hollingshead recalled the encounter, "They thought we were square and we thought they were crazy." The general atmosphere of quietude—the special meditation rooms, the statues of the Buddha, the emphasis on The

101

Tibetan Book of the Dead—was unbearably stuffy to the Pranksters, who dubbed the whole thing "the Crypt Trip." In this scene there was no room for electronics, no guitars or videotapes, no American flags, and well, no freakiness. Kesey was not at all interested in structuring the set and setting of an LSD trip so that a spiritual experience would result. Why did acid require picturesque countryside or a fancy apartment with *objets d'art* to groove on and Bach's Suite in B Minor playing on the stereo? A psychedelic adventure on the bus needed no preconceived spiritual overtones; it could be experienced in the context of a family scene, a musical jam, or a plain old party. The Pranksters thought it was fine just going with the flow, taking acid in the midst of whatever was happening, no matter how disorienting or unusual the situation. It was, after all, a question of style, East Coast versus West Coast. The Merry Pranksters were born in California, starting out as a party of outlandish proportions that evolved into a stoned encounter group on wheels. Kesey, having first turned on to LSD in a government drug testing program, saw the whole phenomenon of grassroots tripping as "the revolt of the guinea pigs." Now that he had taken LSD out of the laboratory and away from the white smocks, any notion of a medically sanitized or controlled psychedelic experience was abhorrent to him. Programming the LSD trip with Tibetan vibes struck him as a romantic retreat, a turning back, submitting to another culture's ideas rather than getting into the uniqueness of the American trip. Kesey the psychedelic populist was attempting to broaden the very nature of the tripping experience by incorporating as many different scenes and viewpoints as possible.[5]

This would also be the first time that spooks got a got look at Kesey and the Pranksters as, unbeknownst to Leary, a few were hanging around anonymously already in Millbrook. But the Pranksters didn't stay for long; they grew rather bored and besides frolicking around in the waterfalls, they were getting homesick and ready to return to California. "When you've got something like we've got," Kesey explained, "you can't just sit on it and possess it, you've got to move off of it and give it to other people. It only works if you bring other people into it."[6] And that's what they did. Upon returning to the Golden State, the Pranksters staged a series of public art gatherings, the Electric Kool-Aid Acid Tests of the mid-1960s, which turned on hundreds of people at a time. Kesey, after getting mixed reviews on his second novel, turned to filmmaking as he set out to edit the rolls of footage from his magic bus ride into a completed movie. Parts of the film were shown during these acid tests; sometimes the Grateful Dead were there providing the on-the-spot soundtrack. Bizarre outfits and strobe lights added color to the technicolor trips. Kesey even turned on Hunter S. Thompson and the notorious biker gang the Hell's Angels in the summer of 1965.

Thompson was following the bikers around and doing research for the book he was writing about them, *Hell's Angels: The Strange and Terrible Saga of the Motorcycle Gangs,* when he invited Kesey to come hang out in Monterey. "We're in the same business," Kesey told one of the Angels as he hit the joint they were passing around. "You break people's bones, I break people's heads."[7] Kesey invited the motorcycle gang to La Honda for a party, and a huge banner stretched across the lawn welcoming the Hell's Angels as they rode up into an endless supply of beer kegs and LSD. The police were on guard nearby with ten squad cars and loads of ammunition, as the neighbors locked their doors and huddled inside while engine roars of Harley Davidsons echoed in the distance. It seemed that everyone was at the party: Ginsberg, Ram Dass, Thompson and scores of Bay Area intellectuals—all mingling with acid tripping members of the Hell's Angels:

> Contrary to certain dire expectations of brutal carnage wreaked by drug-twisted criminals, the LSD made the bikers rather docile. They all walked around in a daze, mingling with the radicals, pacifists, and intellectuals. There was Allen Ginsberg, the epitome of much they despised, a gay New York poet chanting Hare Krishna and dancing with his finger cymbals, and the Angels

were actually digging him. It was quite a spectacle. The befuddled policemen stayed outside the grounds with their red flashers blinking through the trees. With so many of the Angels bombed out of their minds, the cops deemed it wise to keep their distance. The party went on for two days—a monument to what the Pranksters had set out to accomplish on the '64 bus trip. They had broken through the worst hang-up intellectuals have—the "real life" hangup. After this first bash the Angels hung around Kesey's for the next six weeks, attending numerous Prankster parties. Their presence added a certain voltage that was unforgettable for those in attendance.[8]

Hunter Thompson later wished he could repeat those early acid trips in La Honda with the Hell's Angels, writing, "It was a very electric atmosphere. If the Angels lent a feeling of menace, they also made it more interesting... and far more alive than anything likely to come out of a controlled experiment or a politely brittle gathering of well-educated truth-seekers looking for wisdom in a capsule. Dropping acid with the Angels was an adventure; they were too ignorant to know what to expect, and too wild to care."[9]

Kesey's scene, a love-filled acid freakout was all the rage in the Bay Area as a new generation learned new psychological truths from having their minds stretched to the unknown by psychedelic drugs. If you could "pass the Acid Test" then you were free to cut the cords of your parents and everything the older generation had deemed safe and status quo. But to the CIA, these experiments with LSD turned out to be a disaster, as what was once supposed to be a quest for a truth serum turned into an out of control culture with a diaspora all its own that the agency was at a loss to explain. So they moved to contain it. LSD was suddenly declared illegal in 1966, a year after the first big wave of street acid hit the scene. But this did little to dissuade the youth from diving head first into the Abyss. Psychedelics were meant to be liberating, a way to confront your reality in the cosmic drama of life. The world was changing at a rapid rate and LSD was trailblazing the path for a new generation, one that wanted to evolve consciousness, spread love and remove the invisible chains of the establishment slave masters. Kesey retreated back to Oregon and didn't write another novel for decades; the other acid godfather, Timothy Leary, was hounded by The Man and thrown in prison for a few grams of marijuana. By the late 60s, beatnik godfather Kerouac had drunk himself to death down in Florida, the innocence of the 50s was long gone and Vietnam was the first televised war, while the youth of the 60s lived a daily apocalypse full of assassinations, riots and antiwar movements. And as the CIA looked to curtail their failed foray into psychedelics, they had a bigger problem on their hands as the counterculture was now going mainstream thanks to high profile rock stars like Jim Morrison threatening to red pill the masses.

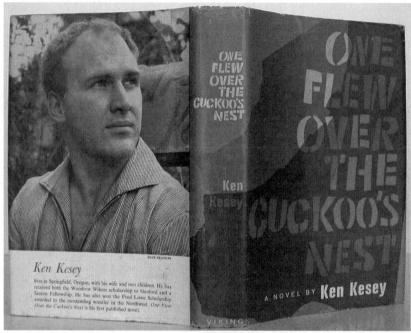

Ken Kesey's landmark first novel (*Pinterest*)

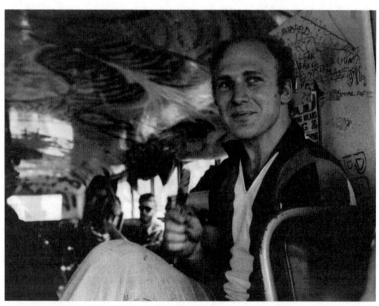

Ken Kesey aboard the Furthur Bus (*Pinterest*)

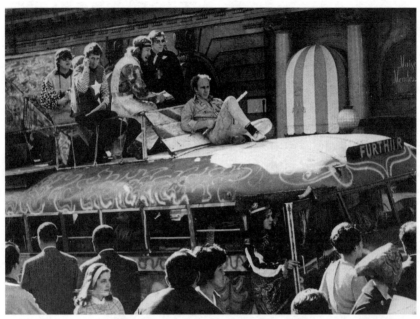

The Merry Pranksters (*Pinterest*)

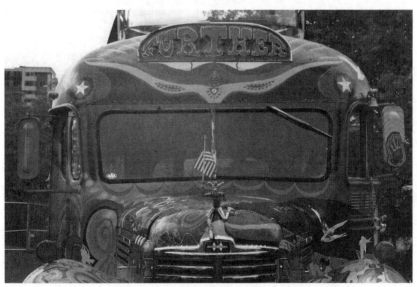

Furthur the Magic Bus (*Wikiwand*)

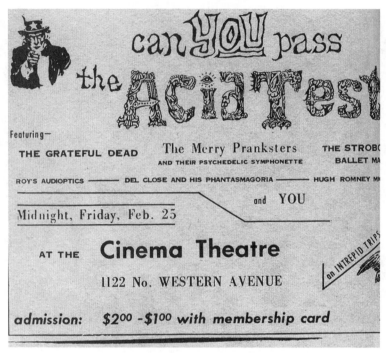

Flyer for an early San Francisco acid test

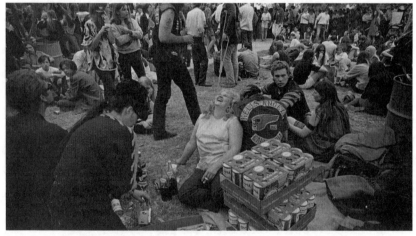

Hippies and Hell's Angels tripping on acid (*Reddit*)

Chapter Six

The MIC, CIA and the
Wizards of Laurel Canyon

*Well, I just got into town about an hour ago. Took a look
around, see which way the wind blow. Where the little girls in
their Hollywood bungalows? Are you a lucky little lady in the
city of light? Or just another lost angel? City of night.*
— The Doors

When we listen to our musical heroes, we believe they truly
know what the world is about and how to rebel against it. But what
if our anti-establishment rebellious rock idols were nothing more
than MK-ULTRA mindcontrol victims? Purposely placed false
prophets designated to be the leaders of the counterrevolution,
but actually serving the real purpose of a revolution in a war on
intelligence, as a culture of intellect and open thought suddenly
became overrun with rampant drug use and longhaired hippies
thanks in part to the spread of acid. This new social experiment,
conceived in the 60s and perfected by the dawn of the new
millennium, was a form of mind science used on the unsuspecting
youth, most prominently through the art of music. This movement
began to spread its message of peace, drugs, and love while the
escalation of the war in Vietnam boomed after the country's most
popular president was slaughtered on national television. This
era, paved by acid, would eventually lead us spiraling down to
our present path of watching mind controlled musical icons enact
ancient satanic rituals, elaborately staged and broadcast in high
definition and surround sound to the delight of our eyes and ears,
unaware that we are being bombarded with occult symbology,
and satanic theologies descended from ancient pagan astro-
archaeological beliefs. The forces behind the record companies
responsible for this are an elite group of super wealthy individuals,
often summed up as 'The Illuminati.' This nefarious cult has
outstretched tentacles that run their business through the occult,

and are the heads of secret societies like the Freemasons and the O.T.O. Members of these organizations hold high-ranking positions in what we refer to as the Military Industrial Complex. The MIC's ultimate goal is to demoralize the youth, and rewire their brains to a point where they have stopped thinking for themselves, thus eliminating any chance for an uprising during the End Game phase of their plans for a New World Order.

With the help of the CIA, the British MI-6 and projects like MK-ULTRA, the music industry created a new batch of idols who promoted drug use, bad behavior and lyrics steeped in satanic symbolism. Eventually music would be turned into nothing more than an ongoing satanic spectacle, where every video and award ceremony is host to occult symbols and rituals. Gone, too, would be any sort of lyrical mastery. No more social commentary, and no chance for some great poet to awaken the sleeping masses. This esoteric conquering of the music industry has many outstretched tentacles, but the brain of the beast lived in the capital of wizards and witches. Emerging from a hidden hilltop enclave high above the City of Angels, occultists and scientists in a secret military base would go on to perfect the art of mind control. In doing so, they created the West Coast rock scene, the hippie movement, the drug culture, gangster rap and the eventual destruction of society. But this secret satanic experiment with the music industry doesn't just include the West Coast, the blues or the Beatles, but reaches back in time to the occult musical worlds of Mozart and Beethoven.

The year 1967 marked the breaking point in the short history of the United States. The dreams of the British scribes Huxley and Orwell, who wrote *Brave New World* and *1984,* were finally being brought into fruition and the long-planned goals of eugenics, chemical and social engineering finally escalated to warfare status against the unsuspecting American youth. Still recovering from the shock of watching the president getting his brains blown out for everyone to see and the worry of getting drafted in some bullshit war, they could also add going to prison for LSD to a long list of totally ungroovy things. The continued presence of invading American troops increased dramatically during the four years after JFK's death, with over 475,000 serving in Vietnam (mostly poor teenagers); pot smoke and nervous tension filled the air at antiwar rallies nationwide. The fabled "Summer of Love" consisting of horny long haired teenagers smoking weed, tripping balls, and grooving to the vibes of the Dead set the stage for pot-friendly musical gatherings and outdoor rock concerts. It was at the first-ever rock festival in Monterey, California, attended by over 100,000 bright-eyed teens, that the CIA would try its most outlandish acid experiment.

The kids and everyone else in attendance were ready to rock 'n' roll and have a good time—never knowing that they were about to be dosed with LSD sprayed from above. To the CIA the real purpose of Monterey Pop wasn't the hours-long rock festival, but the widespread distribution of psychedelics or hallucinogens, such as LSD, to tens of thousands of teenagers. The agency was looking to spark a mass trip and tactfully sprayed mists of LSD on the unsuspecting pop festival crowd from a helicopter. John Phillips, a member of the rock group The Mamas and the Papas and a CIA asset, spearheaded the LSD spectacle that would come to be known as the Monterey Pop festival. Phillips ran the concert, and was in charge of everything from the stage to the sound acoustics. He wanted to make sure the audience would be getting the full-blown effect of the special Monterey experience. Monterey was historic; for the first time young Americans got to witness the sheer explosiveness of a Who performance, and it marked their introduction to rock's reigning guitar god Jimi Hendrix. After watching the greatest drummer of all time, Keith Moon, rip his set and then destroy his drum kit, the amazed crowd watched the rest of the Who smash their equipment and make a mess on the stage. The bar had been raised to near impossible heights. It was just the motivation Jimi Hendrix needed for his American homecoming to be triumphant. With his electrified Fender guitar, Hendrix oozed sex appeal while executing unheard of guitar riffs at a volume that smashed minds and blew out eardrums. The crowd, engulfed by acid, watched with jaws hanging as Hendrix set his guitar on fire in one of the most legendary performances in rock history. There was open drug use everywhere; mysteriously no one was arrested, and the LSD that was sprayed over the crowd led to the biggest collective trip in history.

A year after the Monterey Pop festival put a new era of rock music on the map, tens of thousands came flooding into San Francisco to join the hippies and turn on the mind via LSD. Inspired by the John Phillips-penned hit "San Francisco (Be Sure to Wear Flowers in Your Hair)" which sold over four million copies, this new musical culture was set in motion when strangers with similar backgrounds came together in the hills of Laurel Canyon in Los Angeles. Most shared a family history within the high rankings of the Military Industrial Complex. Some even had royal bloodlines going back to the Old World. These people who gathered at Laurel Canyon would soon provide the faces and sounds of pop culture, influencing their generation and future ones with the music and films created. But just who were these people and from whence did they come? The late Dave McGowan, the man responsible for opening the can of worms on this subject, sets the stage:

> Meanwhile, elsewhere in the world in those early months of 1965, a new 'scene' is just beginning to take shape in the city of Los Angeles. In a geographically and socially isolated community known as Laurel Canyon—a heavily wooded, rustic, serene, yet vaguely ominous slice of LA nestled in the hills that separate the Los Angeles basin from the San Fernando Valley—musicians, singers and songwriters suddenly begin to gather as though summoned there by some unseen Pied Piper. Within months, the 'hippie/flower child' movement will be given birth there, along with the new style of music that will provide the soundtrack for the tumultuous second half of the 1960s.[1]

But the history of Laurel canyon goes far beyond the lore of the Hollywood Hills—since its inception it's been a land of mystery, magic and murder.

The Tongva natives were the original inhabitants of Laurel Canyon, but these ancient settlers of California would all but vanish during the New World invasion. Blood would be spilled without end during war after war for the right to own California. The United States would finally win this battle in 1848, defeating Mexico in an unpopular and controversial battle. In 1850, the city of Los Angeles would be incorporated, and a sprawling new spin on the metropolis would begin to take root. The old landowners were rounded up and one out of ten either lost his land or was reduced to bankruptcy. The more fortunate Spanish or Native rancheros were absorbed into other communities, depending on their wealth or color. A new wave of extermination was begun by American ranchers and miners intent on ridding California of the last of its native population. The US government actually reimbursed bounty hunters (mostly out of work Civil War veterans) for the scalps of murdered Native Americans. One band was hunted down and murdered in Franklin Canyon. During this time, the entire Los Angeles area fell into anarchy as unsuccessful gold hunters, fugitives, disposed Native Americans, ex-soldiers, aspiring farmers, ranchers and speculators, and even German Jewish merchants flooded the area. A severe drought in 1865 put the last of the Spanish rancho owners out of business. Preying on this hapless population were bandits and outlaws who held out in mountain hideaways.

Laurel Canyon's first famous resident was the bandit Tiburcio Vasques, a romantic hero of Native and Mexican resistance. Vasques eluded authorities by hiding out within the vast canyon lands later dubbed the Hollywood Hills. Other Mexican residents resisted the new Anglo powers by resorting to social banditry against the Gringos. In 1856, Juan Flores threatened the southland with a full-scale Mexican revolt. He was hanged in Los Angeles in front of 3,000 spectators. Tiburcio Vasques, a legend in his own time among the Mexican population for his daring feats against the Anglos, was captured and hanged on La Cienega Boulevard. Things eventually calmed down, and the original Spanish ranchos were subdivided in the 1880s. In 1886, the town of Hollywood was established by H.H. Wilcox (his wife gave the town its name) which began the irreversible shift from agriculture to residences to business. Legend has it that H.H. (Harvey) and Ida moved from Topeka, Kansas in 1884, and strolled into Los Angeles on a baggage car carried by two of their finest thoroughbreds. In Los Angeles Harvey formed a real estate company with an associate and began buying up land, planning and paving the streets, and selling welcoming lots to the influx of wealthy voyagers seeking the warm California sun. From H.H. Wilcox's *Wikipedia* page we learn:

> Harvey and Ida had one child, a son named Harry, who died in 1886 at the age of 18 months. Family tradition says that to console themselves over the death of their baby, Harvey and Ida would take buggy rides to the beautiful canyons west of Los Angeles. Harvey purchased one of their favorite areas for $150 per acre, in an agricultural area of fig and apricot orchards. Harvey tried his hand at raising fruit, but failed and decided to subdivide the land, selling lots for $1,000 each.[2]

His wife named the land "Hollywood" after her friends' summer home in Ohio, and the name Hollywood first appears on the Wilcox's map of the subdivided lots, filed in Los Angeles on February 1, 1887. Another theory links the naming of Hollywood to the ancient 'Toyon Holly' plants found in ample strains decorating the hills of southern California. There is even a man who claims to be the father of Hollywood himself. H.J. Whitley is said to have coined the phrase while on a honeymoon with his wife. His wife Gigi's memoirs supposedly verify this, but good luck finding a copy. One thing we do know is that H.J. did have a huge impact on the future of Hollywood; he basically owned all the land it was built upon. Whitley is a conspiracy lover's wet dream; not only was he a successful real estate tycoon—he also owned banks! Whitley was known to socialize with the richest and most powerful people in the world, from presidents to royals. With his monopolistic vision, Hollywood was a thriving community. Prospect Avenue, which would later be called Hollywood Boulevard, was lined with large Queen Anne, Victorian, and Mission Revival houses. Hollywood quickly became a prosperous community by the turn of the century, sporting a post office, a newspaper, a hotel and two markets. Hollywood incorporated in 1903 and celebrated with a parade and automobile race. Several thousand people gathered for the festivities, "Most of them leading citizens from this, and adjoining cities, who had come on personal invitation—800 being taken out on special cars on the trolley line—gathered in the hot sun and listened for hours to speeches on good roads by 'the wizard of Hollywood' H.J. Whitley"[3] and other various members of the early Hollywood elite. This quote from a newspaper published in 1903 is the first reference of an occult or magical term in the history of Hollywood. By referring to Whitley as the 'wizard' of Hollywood we get our first clues to understanding the ongoing spell of Hollywood's enchantment. A history that has its roots not in corny mementos to a friend's summer home or from lovers' lips during a honeymoon, but in ancient sorcery and witchcraft. In the *The Matrix of Power,* prolific occult historian Jordan Maxwell teaches us the real meaning behind Hollywood's origins:

> Merlin and the old magicians of Celtic England always used their magic wands, and these magic wands were always made out of holly-wood. And that's why today we still have Holly-wood, working its "magic" on us — showing us in movies how to view things, what we should think, or just offering us a big box office diversion.[4]

Laurel Canyon provided the perfect backdrop for rich businessmen intent on leaving the smog-filled, claustrophobic cities of the East. The warm sun and ocean breeze was enticing, but the lack of a fresh water supply was a major problem. The desert water riddle was solved by oil baron Edward L. Doheny (Daniel Day Lewis's inspiration for his performance in *There Will Be Blood*) and other land speculators, including H.H. Wilcox and H.J. Whitley, when they teamed up with William Mulholland, a virtuoso hydraulic engineer. In the 2008 *Los Angeles Times* article "Hiking into Hollywood's Backyard," Diane Wedner writes:

> Although oil was plentiful in early 20th century L.A., water was not. Responding to the demand for it, engineer William Mulholland and the Los Angeles Department of Water and Power began construction of the reservoirs in Franklin Canyon in 1914 to distribute water from the Owens Valley to the growing, thirsty region. Their only rival in the water racket would be another key early figure who played a role in developing the canyon, and the

greater Los Angeles area. The real estate tycoon Charles Spencer Mann was a blue blood belonging to one of the oldest families in America. Educated in Chicago he moved west with dreams of building on the unsettled lands of California. Despite the depression and the horrible realty market of the time, Mann found success working at Easton, Eldridge & Co. Assigned Managerial duties this working experience taught Mann all he needed to know about the emerging Los Angeles real estate market. He promptly left the firm in 1902, and established a company of his own.[5]

Realizing the importance of water in the harsh desert climate of southern California, Mann and a few other investors created the Hollywood Water Company. This would fan the flame of inspired purchases around the hills of Hollywood. Mann and his partners began buying up land along what would become Laurel Canyon Boulevard, as well as up Lookout Mountain. A narrow road leading up to the crest of Lookout Mountain was carved out, and upon that crest was constructed a lavish 70-room inn with sweeping views of the city below and the Pacific Ocean beyond. The Lookout Inn featured a large ballroom, riding stables, tennis courts and a golf course, among other amenities. By 1913, Mann began operating what was billed as the nation's first trackless trolley to ferry tourists and prospective buyers from Sunset Boulevard up to what would become the corner of Laurel Canyon Boulevard and Lookout Mountain Avenue. Mann hired local architect Robert Byrd to build Laurel Tavern. Byrd was one of the founding fathers of architecture in Los Angeles. Curiously, the homes he developed within and around Laurel Canyon have witnessed gruesome murders and suicides, with the most famous being the Sharon Tate house on Cielo drive.

Byrd's vision for the Laurel Tavern was extravagant and even included a bowling alley in the basement. Mann eventually sold the property to the famous movie cowboy Tom Mix, who rechristened it simply as the Log Cabin, a name that stuck thanks to Frank Zappa and the future generations who gathered there. Curiously, all these "stars" that would change the culture of the future gathered nearly simultaneously along the narrow, winding

116

roads of Laurel Canyon. They came from across the country as well as from Canada and England to an area where there was no music industry or live music scene at the time—Los Angeles. If you think about it, there was no discernable reason for them to venture to Los Angeles, considering that aspiring musicians in those days went to centers of the musical universes located in Nashville, Memphis and New York. But it wasn't the industry that drew the Laurel Canyon crowd, you see, but rather the Laurel Canyon crowd that transformed Los Angeles into the epicenter of the music industry. To what, then, do we attribute this unprecedented gathering of future musical superstars in the hills above Los Angeles? What Pied Piper inspired them all to head west? Those on the roster of Laurel Canyon superstars are, more often than not, the sons and daughters of the MIC or the sons and daughters of extreme wealth and privilege; oftentimes, you'll find both rolled into one convenient package. And since that link exists with the military, it's safe to say that the boys at the agency were well aware of the blossoming musical scene going on in Laurel Canyon. A scene with its MIC roots in a secret movie studio, the real Hollywood, hidden high above the City of Angels:

> Two ambitious projects in the 1940s brought significant changes to Laurel Canyon. First, Laurel Canyon Boulevard was extended into the San Fernando Valley, providing access to the canyon from both the north and the south. The widened boulevard was now a winding thoroughfare, providing direct access to the Westside from the Valley. Traffic, needless to say, increased considerably, which probably worked out well for the planners of the other project, because it meant that the increased traffic brought about by that other project probably wasn't noticed at all. And that's good, you see, because the other project was a secret one, so if I tell you about it, you have to promise not to tell anyone else. What would become known as Lookout Mountain Laboratory was originally envisioned as an air defense center. Built in 1941 and nestled in two-and-a-half secluded acres off what is now Wonderland Park Avenue, the installation was hidden from view and surrounded

by an electrified fence. By 1947, the facility featured a fully operational movie studio. In fact, it is claimed that it was perhaps the world's only completely self-contained movie studio. With 100,000 square feet of floor space, the covert studio included sound stages, screening rooms, film processing labs, editing facilities, an animation department, and seventeen climate-controlled film vaults. It also had underground parking, a helicopter pad and a bomb shelter. Over its lifetime, the studio produced some 19,000 classified motion pictures—more than all the Hollywood studios combined (which I guess makes Laurel Canyon the real 'motion picture capital of the world'). Officially, the facility was run by the U.S. Air Force and did nothing more nefarious than process AEC footage of atomic and nuclear bomb tests. The studio, however, was clearly equipped to do far more than just process film.

There are indications that Lookout Mountain Laboratory had an advanced research and development department that was on the cutting edge of new film technologies. Such technological advances as 3-D effects were apparently first developed at the Laurel Canyon site. And Hollywood luminaries like John Ford, Jimmy Stewart, Howard Hawks, Ronald Reagan, Bing Crosby, Walt Disney and Marilyn Monroe were given clearance to work at the facility on undisclosed projects. There is no indication that any of them ever spoke of their work at the clandestine studio. The facility retained as many as 250 producers, directors, technicians, editors, animators, etc., both civilian and military, all with top security clearances—and all reporting to work in a secluded corner of Laurel Canyon. Accounts vary as to when the facility ceased operations. Some claim it was in 1969, while others say the installation remained in operation longer. In any event, by all accounts the secret bunker had been up and running for more than twenty years before Laurel Canyon's rebellious teen years, and it remained operational for the most turbulent of those years. The existence of the facility remained unknown to the general public until the early 1990s, though it had long been rumored that the CIA operated a secret movie studio somewhere in or near Hollywood. Filmmaker Peter Kuran was the first to learn of its existence, through classified documents he obtained while researching his 1995 documentary, "Trinity and Beyond." And yet even today, some 15 years after its public disclosure, one would have trouble finding even a single mention of this secret military/intelligence facility anywhere in the 'conspiracy' literature.[6]

Lookout Mountain Laboratory produced more than 6,000 classified films for the Department of Defense and the Atomic Energy Commission, and that's just what we know about; unknown still are all the origin stories for the other odd things that sprang out of Laurel Canyon shortly thereafter. The former top secret studio compound has since been converted into an eight-bedroom, 12-bathroom residence that was purchased by Jared Leto for $5 million in 2015.

But back when the CIA was trying to get a grip on their LSD gone wild experiment there were plenty of spooks posing as entertainers hanging around the canyon scene. There were also spooks who didn't even bother to pose as entertainers streaming into the canyon for top secret work at Lookout Mountain Laboratory at least twenty years before the first rock star appeared upon the scene. Charlton Heston even filmed a series of secret CIA training videos there.[7] A top secret military compound rumored to be the home of CIA black projects just happens to be a rock, skip and a jump away from where all the musical icons of the 60s just sort of spontaneously and serendipitously came together in Laurel Canyon. Sounds too good to be true. But how many strange coincidences do we have to ignore in order to believe that this was just a chance gathering of strangers? What are the odds of arriving in Laurel Canyon and forming a band that finds instant success? And the odds that just a mile down the road from your band lives another guy who recently arrived in Laurel Canyon, who also happens to front a band on the verge of stardom? What if he's married to a girl that you attended kindergarten with, and her dad, like yours, was involved in atomic weapons research and testing? But it gets better, almost every rock star that emerged out of the Canyon scene had families with military intelligence backgrounds from the East Coast, notably the Washington DC and Virginia areas. Although almost all of them hailed from there, they all somehow found themselves on the other side of the country, in an isolated canyon high above Los Angeles, clustered around a top secret military installation just in time for the rise of the counterculture. Coincidence?

> I am gross and perverted/ I'm obsessed 'n deranged/ I have existed for years/ But very little had changed/ I am the tool of the Government/ And industry too/ For I am destined to rule/ And regulate you/ I may be vile and pernicious/ But you can't look away/ I make you think I'm delicious/ With the stuff that I say/ I am the best you can get/ Have you guessed me yet? I am the slime oozin' out from your TV set/ You will obey me while I lead you/ And eat the garbage that I feed you/ Until the day that we don't need you/ Don't go for help...no one will heed you/ Your mind is totally controlled/ It has been stuffed into my mold/ And you will do as you are told/ Until the rights to you are sold.
> —Frank Zappa, *I'm the Slim*

Zappa, the eccentric guitar freak musical genius, was a staunch defender of free speech and in his later years opposed globalism and warned about the dangers of mind control and the unchecked zaniness of the CIA. But during the heyday of the Laurel Canyon scene he was viewed as a father figure. Zappa, curiously enough, never did drugs, save for maybe ten joints that he's claimed to have smoked throughout his lifetime. He hated drugs and believed that the CIA's LSD experiment was designed to prevent youth rebellions and to keep them blitzed out of their minds, unable to see how they were being played for fools. In a magazine article from *Circus Raves* in 1975, Zappa said:

> They were just so full of dope that they were going blindly their own way, not thinking for a moment that the

origin of LSD was in the CIA and a lot of them probably don't like to think about that now. By taking LSD they were helping the CIA in one of their favorite experiments. After they got done taking volunteers from the army, they actually made a profit selling it to people on the street, and seeing what actually happened to a civilian population. They got it in the ass so bad from the CIA that they don't even know. So to sit on the outside of that and say it was stupid will not make you any friends in the group of people who really believe in it, and since there were more of them than of me, it sort of set me up in a negative light for all the years to come. (...) They're a cultural phenomenon, they're an industry, and they're a tool by which the government keeps the kids in check. They also use the same thing to keep the housewives down. Every time you take some dope and you think you're getting some escape from your life, you're just playing right into the government's hand. Every time you use whatever it is that you use, you're registering yourself as a pawn. (...) The minute you start taking those drugs, they got you. I'd rather be free inside of my mind. If you don't have enough money to beat the system, the least you can do is keep your self-respect and know what you think is not chemically induced by a governmental agency.[8]

Words of truth from a man whose father was a chemical scientist for the Air Force. It seems that Zappa knew a lot more than he was supposed to, and although he never obtained the commercial success of his peers, he was still the most influential figure among them:

Ensconced in an abode dubbed the 'Log Cabin'—which sat right in the heart of Laurel Canyon, at the crossroads of Laurel Canyon Boulevard and Lookout Mountain Avenue—Zappa will play host to virtually every musician who passes through the canyon in the mid- to late-1960s. He will also discover and sign numerous acts to his various Laurel Canyon-based record labels. Many of these acts will be rather bizarre and somewhat obscure characters (think Captain Beefheart and Larry "Wild Man" Fischer), but some of them, such as psychedelic rocker cum shock-rocker Alice Cooper, will go on to superstardom. Zappa, along with certain members of his sizable entourage (the 'Log Cabin' was run as an early commune, with numerous hangers-on occupying various rooms in the main house and the guest house, as well as in the peculiar caves and tunnels lacing the grounds of the home; far from the quaint homestead the name seems to imply, by the way, the 'Log Cabin' was a cavernous five-level home that featured a 2,000+ square-foot living room with three massive chandeliers and an enormous floor-to-ceiling stone fireplace), will also be instrumental in introducing the look and attitude that will define the 'hippie' counterculture (although the Zappa crew preferred the label 'Freak'). Nevertheless, Zappa (born, curiously enough, on the Winter Solstice of 1940) never really made a secret of the fact that he had nothing but contempt for the 'hippie' culture that he helped create and that he surrounded himself with... Frank's dad also had little regard for the youth culture of the 1960s, given that Francis Zappa was, in case you were wondering, a chemical warfare specialist assigned to—where else?—the Edgewood Arsenal. Edgewood is, of course, the longtime home of America's chemical warfare program, as well as a facility frequently cited as being deeply enmeshed in MK-ULTRA operations. Curiously enough, Frank Zappa literally grew up at the Edgewood Arsenal, having lived the first seven years of his life in military housing on the grounds of the facility. The family later moved to Lancaster, California, near Edwards Air Force Base, where Francis Zappa continued to busy himself with doing classified work for the military/intelligence complex. His son, meanwhile, prepped himself to become an icon of the peace & love crowd.[9]

One of the first to arrive on the Laurel Canyon scene was Jim Morrison, the enigmatic lead singer of The Doors. With his

Rock God looks and esoteric lyrics Jim quickly become the most controversial, critically acclaimed, and iconic figure to take up residence in Laurel Canyon. The acid gobbling, whiskey swiggin' "Lizard King" was the son of Admiral George Stephen Morrison, the man responsible for the false flag event at the Gulf of Tonkin that led us into the Vietnam War. The Admiral, who was also involved in classified atomic tests at Lookout Mountain, was now assisting to establish a new and illegal war. So, what are the odds that his son would happen to become the spokesperson of the antiwar crowd? Maybe, it's just a small world after all?

Stephen Stills, another early Laurel Canyon star, was a founding member of two of the Canyon's most acclaimed bands— Buffalo Springfield and Crosby, Stills & Nash. Stills also penned the anthem of the 60s "For What It's Worth," a classic protest song against the Vietnam War that actually wasn't. It was inspired by a riot on the Sunset Strip, mostly involving teenagers upset and demonstrating against new curfew laws and the announced closure of their favorite club—Pandora's Box, at 8118 Sunset Boulevard. Pandora's was a small coffee shop that featured poetry readings, folk music and Laurel Canyon bands like Love and Buffalo Springfield. On the night of November 12, 1966, more than two hundred cops squared off against perhaps a thousand kids in an event witnessed by Stills. The LAPD began cracking heads and arresting everyone in sight. Protestors responded by throwing rocks, setting cars ablaze, and attempting to blow up a bus.

One month later, Stills' song commemorating the event would be blasting from radios across the country, signaling the arrival of a new, antiwar generation. Stills later claimed that it wasn't really a protest song and he wanted to make sure he wasn't going to be pigeonholed as some sort of activist, so he ditched writing about protests from there on out. It's safe to say that the media had a good hand in promoting the song as an antiwar piece even though not one word in the lyrics was about Vietnam; instead it was about entitled youth getting triggered and throwing a tantrum because their funhouse got demolished. Stills' follow-up single was entitled "Bluebird" which, coincidentally or not, happened to be the original codename assigned to the MK-ULTRA program, discussed earlier. Before arriving in Laurel Canyon, Stephen Stills was the product of yet another career military family, traveling the world and educated primarily at schools on military bases and elite military academies. At some point Stills ended up in the jungles of Vietnam, at least according to him. His tales, however, would be universally dismissed as drug-induced delusions since Stills arrived on the Laurel Canyon scene at the exact same time the first uniformed troops shipped out. So, of course he didn't serve with uniformed ground troops in Vietnam, but what about all of those "advisers"[10]—CIA/Special Forces who operated in the country years before the arrival of the first official troops? If the CIA did create the counterculture then why not help one of their own soldiers become an icon of the peace generation? Another Laurel Canyon musical icon was David Crosby, the heavily 'stached walrus-looking founding member of the Byrds, and obviously, Crosby, Stills & Nash:

> Crosby is, not surprisingly, the son of an Annapolis graduate and WWII military intelligence officer, Major Floyd Delafield Crosby. Like others in this story, Floyd Crosby spent much of his post-service time traveling the world. Those travels landed him in places like Haiti, where he paid a visit in 1927, when the country just happened to be, coincidentally of course, under military occupation by the U.S. Marines...But David Crosby is much more than just the son of Major Floyd Delafield Crosby. David Van Cortlandt Crosby, as it turns out, is a scion of the closely intertwined Van Cortlandt, Van Schuyler and Van Rensselaer families. And while you're probably thinking, "the Van Who families?," I can assure you that if you plug those names in over at Wikipedia, you can spend a pretty fair amount of time reading up on the power wielded by this clan for the last, oh, two-and-a-quarter centuries or so. Suffice to say that the Crosby family tree includes a truly dizzying array of US senators and congressmen, state senators and assemblymen, governors, mayors, judges, Supreme Court justices, Revolutionary and Civil War generals, signers of the Declaration of Independence, and members of the Continental Congress. It also includes, I

should hasten to add—for those of you with a taste for such things—more than a few high-ranking Masons. Stephen Van Rensselaer III, for example, reportedly served as Grand Master of Masons for New York. And if all that isn't impressive enough, according to the New England Genealogical Society, David Van Cortlandt Crosby is also a direct descendant of 'Founding Fathers' and Federalist Papers' authors Alexander Hamilton and John Jay. If there is, as many believe, a network of elite families that has shaped national and world events for a very long time, then it is probably safe to say that David Crosby is a bloodline member of that clan (which may explain, come to think of it, why his semen seems to be in such demand in certain circles—because, if we're being honest here, it certainly can't be due to his looks or talent). If America had royalty, then David Crosby would probably be a Duke, or a Prince, or something similar (I'm not really sure how that shit works). But other than that, he is just a normal, run-of-the-mill kind of guy who just happened to shine as one of Laurel Canyon's brightest stars.[11]

Whether manufactured or not the hippie movement arrived like a thunderbolt upon the consciousness of America, seen by history as a spontaneous, organic response to the war in Vietnam and the prevailing social conditions of the time. However, it seems that the musicians themselves and various other leaders and founders of the movement were part of the intelligence community and used by the CIA, who were now discrediting and marginalizing the blooming antiwar movement and creating fake opposition strawmen (hippies) that could be easily controlled and led astray, thanks mostly to the widespread distribution of LSD. With this new counterculture seemingly under control the CIA could advance its own agendas under the continued guise of anonymity. Meanwhile across the Atlantic, the MI6 were having their own generational upheavals as their experiments with LSD led to the rise of the Beatles, the first rock band to use the drug to culture shattering effect.

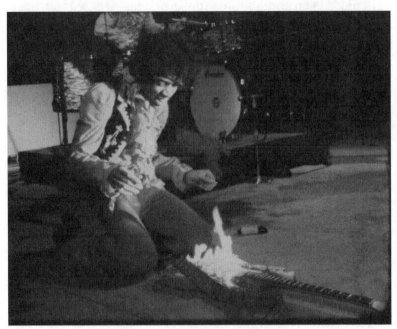

Hendrix and his flaming guitar at the Monterey Pop Festival, 1967
(*Les Paul Forum*)

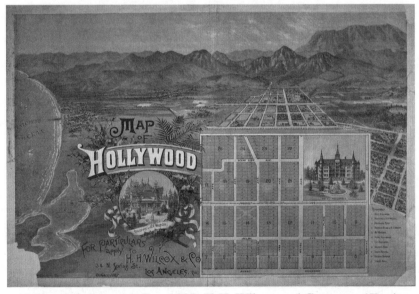

Map of Hollywood, Oct. 1887, H.H. Wilcox and Company (*Kcet*)

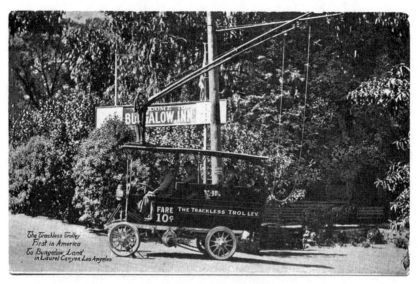

Trackless Trolley (*Kcet*)

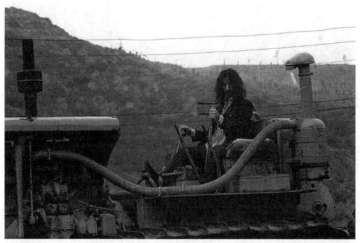

American composer and musician Frank Zappa near his home in
Laurel Canyon (*Mouche Gallery*)

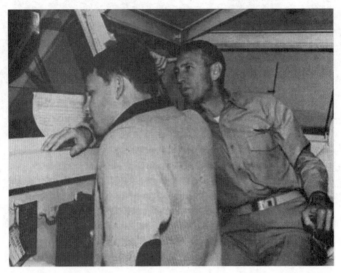

A young Jim Morrison with his Admiral Father (*Business Insider*)

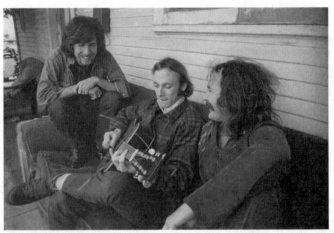

Crosby, Stills & Nash in Laurel Canyon 1969 (*Pinterest*)

Chapter Seven

The MI6, The Beatles and LSD

His hair has the long Jesus Christ look. He is wearing the costume clothes. But most of all, he now has a very tolerant and therefore withering attitude toward all those who are still struggling in the old activist political ways ...while he, with the help of psychedelic chemicals, is exploring the infinite regions of human consciousness.
—Tom Wolfe, *The Electric Kool-Aid Acid Test*

It was spring 1965, in the London suburb of Surrey where John Lennon and his wife, Cynthia, and George Harrison and his wife, Pattie Boyd, were attending a dinner at the home of dentist John Riley when they had their first trip. It wasn't planned but came as a sucker punch from their host who slipped them LSD-laced sugar cubes in their after dinner coffee. Riley urged them to finish their cups and shortly after told Lennon he had placed the LSD sugar cubes in the coffee. Lennon couldn't believe it; he was furious. "How dare you fucking do this to us?" He began to panic. All he knew about the drug was that it caused incredible hallucinations. Lennon's wife also began to freak out after discovering she had been dosed; "It was as if we suddenly found ourselves in the middle of a horror film. The room seemed to get bigger and bigger."[1] The Lennons and Harrisons fled Riley's home in George's Mini Cooper, and they drove off towards Leicester Square's Ad Lib club. In the elevator, their trip got bad. "We all thought there was a fire in the lift," Lennon told *Rolling Stone* in 1971. "It was just a little red light, and we were all screaming, all hot and hysterical."[2] Once inside the club, and isolated away at a table, something like a revelation began to take hold as George Harrison suddenly felt close with the creator of the universe. Later recalling to *Rolling Stone* about his first acid trip, he said, "I had such an overwhelming feeling of well-being, that there was a God, and I could see him in every blade of grass. It was like gaining hundreds of years of experience in 12 hours."[3]

After the club, the couples ended up at the Harrisons' home in Esher, outside of London, where John recalled, "God, it was just terrifying, but it was fantastic. George's house seemed to be just like a big submarine...It seemed to float above his wall, which was 18 foot, and I was driving it. I did some drawings at the time, of four faces saying, 'We all agree with you.' I was pretty stoned for a month or two."[4] A few months later, the Beatles were on their second tour of America where John and George decided to take LSD again on their own terms during time off in Los Angeles. Their proper introduction to LSD would take place, of course, near Laurel Canyon, where the band holed up for a psychedelics party in Zsa Zsa Gabor's house with Peter Fonda and David Crosby. The date of this infamous ordeal was August 24, 1965, the location was 2850 Benedict Canyon in Beverly Hills, the outcome changed popular music forever. A day of good vibes, bad vibes, death vibes, sex vibes, swimming and songs, ideas for new tunes and cool actors that weren't so cool. It was a momentous day for the band...

George Harrison: John and I had decided that Paul and Ringo had to have acid because we couldn't relate to them anymore. Not just on the one level, we couldn't relate to them on any level because acid had changed us so much.

John Lennon: We just decided to take LSD again on tour in 1965, in one of those houses, like Doris Day's house, or wherever it was we used to stay...

George Harrison: It was a horseshoe-shaped house on a hill off Mulholland.

John Lennon: It was something out of Disneyland.

Peter Fonda: The Beatles stayed on Benedict Canyon in a stilt house. I was asked to come over and I went in my Jag. I had been instructed to give a password to the police who were guarding the house, but the reason for such protection only sank in when I came to a bend in the road, just before their rented house, and saw that the entire wall of the canyon was filled with screaming young people.

John Lennon: We just took it, Ringo, George and I, and Neil Aspinall and a couple of the Byrds, what's his name? The one in the Stills and Nash thing? Crosby, and the other guy, who used to do the lead, McGuinn.

George Harrison: But Paul wouldn't have LSD; he didn't want it. So Ringo and Neil took it, while Mal stayed straight in order to take care of everything. Dave Crosby and Roger McGuinn of the Byrds had also come up, and I don't know how, but Peter Fonda was there.

Peter Fonda: As soon as I was in the house, David Crosby gave me my "dose" of LSD.

George Harrison: I had a concept of what had happened the first time I took LSD, but the concept is nowhere near as big as the reality when it actually happens. So as it kicked in again, I thought, "Jesus, I remember!" I was trying to play the guitar, and then I got in the swimming pool, and it was a great feeling; the water felt good.

John Lennon: We were in the garden, it was only our second time doing LSD, and we still didn't know anything about doing it in a nice place, and cool it, and all that... we just took it. And all of a sudden we saw the reporter, Don Short, and we're thinking, "How do we act normal?" Because we imagined we were acting extraordinary, which we weren't. We thought, "Surely somebody can see?"

George Harrison: I was swimming across the pool when I heard a noise, because it makes your senses so acute, you can almost see out of the back of your head. I felt this bad vibe, and I turned around and it was Don Short from *The Daily Mirror*. He'd been hounding us all through the tour, pretending in his phony-baloney way to be friendly, but was really trying to nail us.

John Lennon: We were terrified waiting for Don Short to go, and Neil Aspinall, who had never had acid either, had taken it, and still had to play road manager, so we said to him, "Go get rid of Don Short..."

George Harrison: We were in one spot, John and me and Roger McGuinn, and Don Short, who was probably only about 20 yards away, talking. But it was as though we were looking through the wrong end of a telescope. And Don seemed to be in the very far distance, and we were saying, "Oh fuck, there's that guy over there..." Neil had to take him to play pool, trying to keep him away.

Ringo Starr: Neil had to deal with Don Short while I was swimming in jelly in the pool.

Don Short: Neil Aspinall escorted me downstairs to the pool room, because I was the only journalist on the premises. His job was to divert my attention from the fact that everyone else was taking acid.

George Harrison: LSD's definitely not the kind of drug you'd want to be playing pool with Don Short on.

George Harrison: Fonda kept saying, "I know what it's like to be dead, because I shot myself." He'd accidentally shot himself at some time, and he was showing us his bullet wound.

Peter Fonda: When I was ten years old, I'd accidentally shot myself in the stomach, and my heart stopped beating three times while I was on the operating table because I'd lost so much blood.

John Lennon: Peter Fonda kept sitting next to me, and whispering, "I know what it's like to be dead...." We were saying, "For chrissakes, shut up, we don't care! We don't want to know!"

George Harrison: Fonda was very uncool.

Ringo Starr: It was a fabulous day. The night wasn't so great, because it felt like it was never going to wear off. 12 hours later, and it was, "Give us a break now, Lord..."[5]

Acid, ultimately transformed everything about the Beatles—their sound, their confidence, their ideas and their influence on history. However, McCartney, the squarest of the bunch, declined to trip with his bandmates and Lennon and Harrison never forgot his refusal or forgave him. For Lennon LSD was a third eye opener, understood better by him after reading *The Psychedelic Experience: A Manual Based on the Tibetan Book of the Dead* by Timothy Leary, Ralph Metzner and Richard Alpert (Ram Dass).

The authors, who had researched psychedelics for both therapeutic and mystical purposes, were the same ones that Kesey and his band of Pranksters couldn't stand to be around in Millbrook. But their adaptation of an eighth-century Buddhist book as a primer to killing your ego through the psychedelic experience was a godsend to Lennon. With passages like, "Do not cling in fondness and weakness to your old self. Even though you cling to your old mind, you have lost the power to keep it. Trust your divinity, trust your brain, and trust your companions. Whenever in doubt, turn off your mind, relax, float downstream." Lennon now had a frame of reference to make sense of what the drug did to him and his artistic inspiration.

Within days, Lennon presented a new Beatles song to producer George Martin that began, "Turn off your mind, relax and float downstream/It is not dying, it is not dying/Lay down all thoughts, surrender to the void/It is shining, it is shining,"[6] a vision of the eerie transmigration of the soul scored by LSD. The song, "Tomorrow Never Knows," would become the Beatles first LSD-inspired tune, and while other bands—the Grateful Dead, Jefferson Airplane, Quicksilver Messenger Service, The Doors and Pink Floyd—all made music in extended improvisation passages while tripping, the Beatles were smart and good enough not to need any extra psychedelic inspiration during the recording process. "We found out very early," Ringo Starr said, "that if you play it stoned or derelict in any way, it was really shitty music, so we would have the experiences and then bring that into the music later."[7]

With Lennon's "Tomorrow Never Knows" setting the standard for *Revolver*; the Beatles kicked off the era of psychedelic sound bombings that saw them recording in an amazing array of styles, most of which were newly invented and entirely new to pop music. After their acid initiation Lennon and Harrison became a lot tighter as George later recalled: "After taking acid together, John and I had a very interesting relationship. John and I spent a lot of time together from then on and I felt closer to him than all the others, right through until his death. As Yoko came into the picture, I lost a lot of personal contact with John; but on the odd occasion I did see him, just by the look in his eyes, I felt we were connected."[8] That connection was highlighted during the last recording session for *Revolver*, that saw Lennon's Peter Fonda disk track "She Said She Said" get recorded without Paul. McCartney made suggestions that Lennon rejected and a war of insults and "fuck offs" ensued as Lennon made sure the track was one of the only Beatles songs Paul never played on. John's real reason, and George and Ringo understood this, was that since Paul didn't trip on acid with the rest of them, he didn't deserve to take part in the Peter Fonda diss record. For the band, it was a breach that never truly healed, and it prefigured greater divisions to come, when Lennon, Harrison and Starr all aligned against McCartney all the way through legal suits—and the breakup of the Beatles, the greatest band ever. But not before they continued their streak of LSD inspired albums, including their follow up to *Revolver*, the mind-bending masterpiece *Sgt. Pepper's Lonely Hearts Club Band*. A cultural landmark that changed music forever when released, *Sgt. Pepper's* was immediately hailed as the greatest artistic achievement of the Beatles' career, a shocking move from a once clean-cut band used to churning out lovey dovey pop tunes. With a whole new look and no longer thought of aspassé—the Beatles thrust their psychedelic imaginations upon the world. A world forever altered by music and LSD. Acid visionary Timothy Leary said:

> The *Sgt. Pepper* album… compresses the evolutionary development of musicology and much of the history of Eastern and Western sound in a new tympanic complexity. Then add psychedelic drugs. Millions of kids turned-on pharmacologically, listening to stoned-out electronic music designed specifically for the suggestible, psychedelecized nervous system by stoned-out, long-haired minstrels. This… is the most powerful brainwashing device our planet has ever known. Indeed, if you were an observer from a more highly evolved planet wondering how to change human psychology and human cultural development… would you not inevitably combine electrical energies from outside with biochemical catalysts inside to accomplish your mutation?[9]

McCartney would eventually take LSD once without the company of the other Beatles and went on to make a bunch of unbearable records with a band called Wings, giving hope to the rumors that the original Paul died in the 1960s and was replaced by Billy Shears. Lennon was later murdered by the deep state for knowing way too much about everything, including the CIA's role in introducing LSD to the youth and making it hip via the same music Lennon was guilty of producing. If the CIA were instrumental in using certain Laurel Canyon bands to help create the counterculture in the west, then it's safe to say that the MI6 had a leash on the Beatles too, as the band was the single greatest tool for change in British social engineering efforts. A fact Lennon alluded to in a 1972 interview: "Changing the lifestyle and appearance of youth throughout the world didn't just happen—we set out to do it. We knew what we were doing."[10]

It would be an extremely rare thing if the British Psychological Warfare Division and other intelligence agencies weren't actively behind the promotion of the Beatles, since their music played a key role in a mass social experiment that changed the course of history. Lennon even admitted to *Playboy* that the Beatles were part of a massive social experiment used by Tavistock and other intelligence agencies to introduce drugs like LSD into the mushrooming counterculture scene during the 1960s and 1970s. Even though Lennon benefitted from the drug, he couldn't understand why it flooded the streets just before becoming illegal, and figured the rise of LSD had a way more clandestine origin, correctly calling out the CIA for its misuse of the drug.

> Playboy: Acid?
>
> Lennon: Not in years. A little mushroom or peyote is not beyond my scope, you know, maybe twice a year or something. You don't hear about it anymore, but people are still visiting the cosmos. We must always remember to thank the CIA and the Army for LSD. That's what people forget. Everything is the opposite of what it is, isn't it, Harry? So get out the bottle, boy…and relax. They invented LSD to control people and what they did was give us freedom. Sometimes it works in mysterious ways

its wonders to perform. If you look in the Government reports on acid, the ones who jumped out the window or killed themselves because of it, I think even with Art Linkletter's daughter, it happened to her years later. So, let's face it, she wasn't really on acid when she jumped out the window. And I've never met anybody who's had a flashback on acid. I've never had a flashback in my life and I took millions of trips in the Sixties.[11]

LSD, in combination with psychedelic music made people easier to control and manipulate as the masses that turned on and tuned out couldn't effectively resist other agendas of the deep state such as the ever-expanding war machine in Southeast Asia. The region was a gold mine for defense contractors and future opium dealers, as mass LSD consumption went extinct in favor of far more damaging drugs like heroin and crack cocaine. With the counterculture steered the way the CIA wanted, eventually the music died and most of the rock stars of the era died along with it. The antiwar movement was rendered impotent, and the deep state had over a decade to gather up all the illegal resources needed for full spectrum dominance in the decades to come. As for the British experiments with LSD, they weren't as heavy as what the Americans were doing, but the MI6 still carried out a series of acid tests that wouldn't see the light of day for decades:

Eric Gow was told he was helping to find a cure for the common cold. In fact he was being dosed with LSD in chemical warfare trials. Fifty years on, he and other guinea pigs want to know the truth behind the secret experiments. Eric Gow had a vivid experience when he was aged 19, something that he will never forget. He found that he could not add up three numbers. The radiator in the room started to go in and out "like a squeezebox", shoe-marks on the floor spun around "like a catherine wheel firework". In the evening, he was still tripping—he saw brightly coloured images in the phonebooth as he was calling for a taxi. Eric was not some hippie in search of a magical higher consciousness. He was a serving member of Britain's armed forces in a top-secret military laboratory, who had been ordered to drink a colourless liquid by scientists. He and other young men were being used as human guinea pigs in highly classified experiments directed, it seems, by Britain's spies. According to new evidence uncovered by the Guardian, MI5 and MI6 subjected the men to LSD without telling them what they were doing. The men say they were duped—allegations being investigated by police as part of a two-year inquiry into the use of humans in chemical warfare trials. In the depths of the cold war British intelligence, in collaboration with the CIA, were keen to find out if LSD could be used as a truth drug during interrogations. But even today the guinea pigs are finding it difficult to get the government to admit these psychedelic experiments took place.[12]

CIA documents revealed that in 1951, British intelligence officials agreed to cooperate with the agency in its LSD research, however the documents detailing the British end of this cooperation remained hidden, with the Brits only admitting that 136 servicemen were tested with LSD at Porton between 1961 and 1968, for a military program that had nothing to do with the MI6. But Peter Wright, the MI5 officer and scientist who fought Margaret Thatcher and the British government for the right to publish his memoirs, *Spycatcher,* revealed, "The whole area of chemical research was an active field in the 1950s. I was co-operating with MI6 in a joint programme to investigate how far the hallucinatory drug LSD could be used in interrogations, and extensive trials took place at Porton. I even volunteered as a guinea pig on one occasion."[13]

Documents buried deep in declassified vaults corroborate Wright's statement, as British intelligence was also worried about youth rebellions, Russian spies and if there were any truth serum drugs that could be used on captured insurgents. A document from 1965 revealed that Dr. Bill Ladell, then in charge of human experiments at Porton, had known that "previous trials on LSD had been carried out at Porton many years before, but these had been tentative and inadequately controlled." And Ladell would know, as according to Wright, he "handled all MI5 and MI6 work"[14] at Porton. Despite the government's insistence to deny any involvement regarding MI5 and MI6 operations on LSD research, we know that, "there was, in fact, research being carried out at Porton Down involving LSD, as early as 1953"[15] marking the same time that these acid tests were being conducted by the CIA in America. After keeping the trials secret for decades, the MI6 agreed to pay their former test subjects financial compensation in 2006. Like the CIA, MI6 decided that LSD was not a practical drug for brainwashing or truth serum purposes and was far too powerful an agent acting to break the mind control and help spread the truth about the false matrix of reality most are imprisoned in. For this reason, any future mass social experiments in psychedelics would become non-existent as the drugs became illegal, and shunned to the point where they simply disappeared at a mass level. By becoming a mystic relic of your grandparents' era, LSD and the tales associated with it would become shelved on dusty bookcases and read as fantastic works of fiction. Like the tale of when the CIA helped the French Air Force drop bombs laced with LSD on Pont-Saint-Esprit, a sleepy little village in southern France.

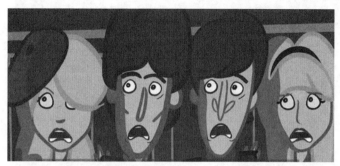

Lennon, Harrison and their wives' first acid trip (*Nerdist*)

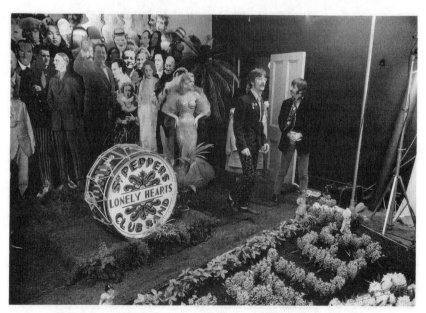

Rare behind the scenes look at the photo shoot for the Sgt. Peppers album cover (*Diana Dors*)

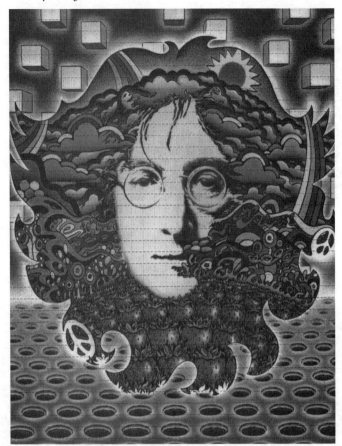

John Lennon acid blotter art (*Jeff Hopp*)

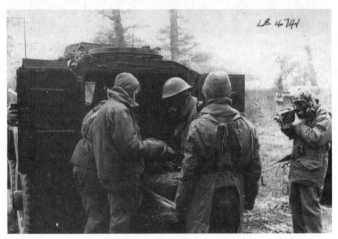

When the British army tried LSD (*Force TV*)

Chapter Eight

LSD Over Pont-Saint-Esprit and the Rise of Psychedelic Cinema

Every record has been destroyed or falsified, every book rewritten, every picture has been repainted, every statue and street building has been renamed, every date has been altered. And the process is continuing day by day and minute by minute. History has stopped. Nothing exists except an endless present in which the Party is always right.
—George Orwell, *1984*

The mystery of where the LSD came from that rocked the French town of Pont-Saint-Esprit, in the Gard, southeast France, over fifty years ago has long been a fascinating tale buried among the classified LSD adventure stories of the CIA. Was it sprayed from above during a secret Air Force flyover? Sprayed from aerosol cans like graffiti taggers in the Bronx? Or cooked into some good ol' fashioned French bread? The 'cursed bread' left residents of the village suffering hallucinations, as the whole town seemed to be experiencing a mass trip. This wouldn't be out of range for the CIA, who once considered dropping LSD into an entire city's water supply. A sleepy little town in Southern France? Surely no one would notice. The CIA, along with the US Army's top secret Special Operations Division (SOD), were able to get some of the good psychedelic stuff from the scientists at Sandoz Pharmaceutical Company, who were already secretly supplying both the Army and CIA with LSD, as we discussed earlier. CIA documents pertaining to the suspicious suicide of Frank Olson, a

141

biochemist working for the CIA who fell from a 13th floor window two years after the mass trip in France, point out conversations between a CIA agent and a Sandoz official who mentions the "secret of Pont-Saint-Esprit."[1] Explaining that it wasn't caused by mold but by diethylamide, the D in LSD, the Sandoz official was basically admitting the acid had something to do with the event. While compiling the book *A Terrible Mistake: The Murder of Frank Olson and the CIA's Secret Cold War Experiments*, the author spoke to Frank Olson's former colleagues, two of whom told him that the Pont-Saint-Esprit incident was part of a mind control experiment run by the CIA and US Army.

LSD was used on unsuspecting troops after the Korean War, as the Army launched a vast research program into the mental manipulation of prisoners and enemy troops. These programs also targeted small towns and out of the way villages where nobody would really notice outside of fifty miles. There was no Internet then. The author learned that CIA agents had sprayed LSD into the air, and just in case that wasn't enough, they also contaminated the local food products of Pont-Saint-Esprit. A White House document sent to members of the Rockefeller Commission to investigate CIA abuses contained the names of French nationals who had been secretly employed by the CIA and were directly involved in the Pont Saint Esprit event. But in their quest to research LSD as a weapon, the Army also drugged over 6,000 unwitting American servicemen between 1953 and 1965. No records indicate whether the French secret service were aware or involved in the alleged operation, and they have come out recently against the CIA, demanding to know whether they dropped LSD on Pont-Saint-Esprit or not. The CIA were heavily interested in knowing if LSD could control a popular revolt, and a mass hallucination on an unsuspecting town was up their alley as far as experimentation goes.

Charles Granjoh, 71, a survivor of the French mass trip still has nightmares from the terrifying ordeal. "I almost kicked the bucket," he told the weekly French magazine *Les Inrockuptibles*. "I'd like to know why." Perhaps, the CIA should tell him that in 1951, his quiet, picturesque village in southern France was suddenly and mysteriously turned into a mess of mass insanity and hallucinations thanks to the LSD they dropped on it. This wasn't a quiet affair. At least five people died, animals went nuts and dozens were interned in insane asylums as hundreds of townsfolk were afflicted. The mystery of Le Pain Maudit (Cursed Bread) still haunts the inhabitants of Pont-Saint-Esprit old enough to remember frightful hallucinations of fire-breathing dragons:

> One man tried to drown himself, screaming that his belly was being eaten by snakes. An 11-year-old tried to strangle his grandmother. Another man shouted: "I am a plane", before jumping out of a second-floor window, breaking his legs. He then got up and carried on for 50 yards. Another saw his heart escaping through his feet and begged a doctor to put it back. Many were taken to the local asylum in strait jackets. *Time* magazine wrote at the time: "Among the stricken, delirium rose: patients thrashed wildly on their beds, screaming that red flowers were blossoming from their bodies, that their heads had turned to molten lead." Eventually, it was determined that the best-known local baker had unwittingly contaminated his flour with ergot, a hallucinogenic mold that infects rye grain.[2]

For nearly 60 years, the Pont-Saint-Esprit incident has been attributed to either ergot poisoning, meaning that the villagers consumed bread infected with a psychedelic mold, or to organic mercury poisoning, but it's safe to say at this point what the real culprit was—LSD. Even the scientists at the British Medical Journal concluded that mold couldn't explain the mass trip that struck hundreds of people in the village. But scientists dispatched to the scene from the Sandoz Chemical company in nearby Basel, Switzerland, covered their and the CIA's tracks by quickly stating that ergot-infused moldy bread was the cause of the trip and there's nothing more to see here; move along. It definitely wasn't a top secret CIA experiment known as Operation Span, conducted under Project MK-NAOMI, a cousin of the more notorious MKULTRA—was it? The 1951 Pont-Saint-Esprit outbreak was the result of a covert LSD aerosol experiment directed by the CIA, and the bogus cover-up was the contaminated bread story. The 'cursed bread' tale was given to the media so they wouldn't know that the Sandoz Pharmaceutical Company, which was then secretly supplying both the US Army and CIA with LSD for research, was involved.

The media also never knew that a year prior to the Pont St. Esprit LSD experiment, the CIA had targeted New York City's subway system for a similar experiment. An FBI memo from 1950 read, "[The] BW [biological warfare] experiments to be conducted by representatives of the Department of the Army in the New York Subway System in September, 1950, have been indefinitely postponed."[3] The memo went on to cite the FBI's concerns about "poisoning of food plants" and the "poisoning of the water supply" of large cities; clearly the feds should have been keeping an eye on the CIA instead of pot smoking hippies. Speaking of which, the psychedelic scene back on the West Coast wasn't just having an effect on music, it was also breaking the long-held power of mainstream movie houses controlling the flow of the film industry. With sudden independent movie hits like *Easy Rider*, the landscape had changed as the rise of psychedelic-fueled independent film companies became commercially and critically successful.

Peter Fonda, Hollywood royalty and cult hero actor of *Easy Rider,* rode the gravy train of cool after starring in one of the most influential films in Hollywood history. The rise of the hippie generation and LSD collided at the crossroads of the film industry, where the old Hollywood system had become stagnant and a bore while young filmmakers experimenting with psychedelics were revitalizing the medium, making films that were having a real impact on the culture and their generation. *Easy Rider* was the movie that broke the mold of the industry, marking a turning point in American cinema and the way movies were made in Hollywood. The independent movie was shot with a budget of $550,000 but went on to gross over $60 million at the box office in 1969:

It was shot outside the studio in real locations over a seven week period, much of the dialogue and narrative were improvised, it featured no major stars and cast nonprofessional actors in several key scenes, it prefigured the MTV generation by twelve years with its inclusion of numerous music video-like vignettes featuring popular rock songs, and it presented an authentic view of the counterculture from inside it because the young cast and crew were a part of it. They were the new Hollywood rebels.[4]

Earning two Oscar nominations, the film went on to become a landmark visual portrait of the counterculture era. It was inspired during Peter Fonda's promotional tour for the world's first LSD movie, the Roger Corman vehicle *The Trip*. LSD movies were all about the visuals, and filmmakers of the era had a helluva time trying to translate that experience onto film without unintended hilarious effects. At least Director Roger Corman dropped acid before he made *The Trip* for authenticity, much like Otto Preminger tripped with Timothy Leary before filming *Skidoo!* which turned out exactly how you'd expect. Save for the iconic *Easy Rider*, most films of the psychedelic era were horrible, didn't make any money and have been mostly forgotten. But thanks to Youtube and nostalgia for the hippie era, we can still watch some of those lost gems of psychedelic cinema. Below are the films that will take you back to the era of free love, acid, bell bottoms, drug awareness educational videos and vomit-inducing strobe lights.

The Tingler (1959)

Vincent Price was one of the first actors to trip on film in this B-movie horror flick about a doctor investigating the roots of fear, who shoots up LSD and dictates his experience into a tape recorder. The film mimics the CIA's blatant anti-LSD propaganda that would emerge in the years after its release, while inadvertently blowing the whistle that they were the ones supplying the doctors in the first place.

The Trip (1967)

Peter Fonda practices for his role in *Easy Rider* by playing a television commercial director with girl troubles who decides to experiment with LSD. Written by Jack Nicholson, the film is basically a summary of his divorce and how he used LSD treatments with a shrink to deal with it. Bruce Dern plays the shrink for Fonda's journey of self-discovery, but when Fonda starts tripping he runs from the couch and goes out into nightclubs, a laundromat and other groovy Southern California locations. The Trip was very pro-LSD, and psychedelic culture in general; it tried to present the therapeutic and medical benefits of the drug as opposed to demonizing it, which makes sense because the major players behind the film—Jack Nicholson, Peter Fonda and Dennis Hopper were all experienced acid heads.

Psych-Out (1968)
Dick Clark produced this disaster of a movie that starred Susan Strasberg as a 17-year-old deaf runaway looking for her brother in Haight-Ashbury at the height of the hippie era. She runs into the usual band of clichéd hippies including the pony-tailed guitar playing Stoney (Jack Nicholson) and Dave (Dean Stockwell) the homeless mistreated war veteran. When they finally find her brother (Bruce Dern), an acid gobbling holy man living at the city dump, they manage to save him, but not before someone depressingly dies near the Golden Gate Bridge.

Wild in The Streets (1968)
This mind-blowing satire stars Christopher Jones, a James Dean lookalike who burned out shortly after filming, playing a messianic rock star who becomes President of the United States. He puts his mother (Shelley Winters) in an acid concentration camp while Richard Pryor takes a page out of the CIA's playbook and doses Washington DC's water supply.

Riot on Sunset Strip (1967)
Filmed during the actual teen riots on the strip, with footage incorporated into the movie about a police captain trying to keep the peace on the streets while his rebellious daughter trips on LSD while exploring the neon Neverland of nighttime Los Angeles.

The Hallucination Generation (1966)
This cheesy film stars medallion wearing George Montgomery

146

as a self-styled guru, amateur chemist, and aspiring acid dealer who gathers kids at his swinging bachelor pad and slips them mickeys of LSD in their drinks. The young acidhead drifters under his influence become hip to a life of crime, complete with psychedelic sequences that will have you scratching your head in disbelief that such a film was ever made.

The Big Cube (1969)
Lana Turner trips in this howler about a famous stage actress whose daughter conspires to drug her mom with LSD in order to drive her insane and inherit her money.

Mantis in Lace (1968)
This bizarre film about a psychotic go-go dancer who murders men in an abandoned warehouse while freaked out on LSD was shot by award winning cinematographer Laszlo Kovacs (*Easy Rider*) and features psychedelic sequences too outrageous even for the era.

Skidoo (1968)
Otto Preminger's counterculture LSD musical mess about turning on old people should be enough to scare you away from drugs forever.

Go Ask Alice (1973)
The most popular "drugs are bad m'kay" movie produced in the hippie era, and yet another negative depiction of the LSD experience committed to film, is this made-for-TV special based on the popular yet fake tales from a teenage girl's diary. Teenagers of the time were constantly bombarded with anti-drug propaganda and silly little shows like *Go Ask Alice*, and as a result most dove into the acid experience with preconceived views of negativity, usually ending in a freak out or bad trip. In fact, most bad trips were just the common outcomes of bad pre-programming thanks to the media, where so-called educational films kept people in the dark about psychedelics drugs instead of teaching them how to take them properly and responsibly.

147

LSD: Insight or Insanity (1966)

Another classic educational film about LSD, hosted by Laurel Canyon murder alumni Sal Mineo, who narrates this slice of 60s teen pie. One of the many anti-LSD school documentaries that were shown in classrooms across the country in an attempt to scare kids away from trying it.

The anti-LSD films broadcast on the American airwaves in the hippie era probably did more harm than good by promoting misinformation and outright lies about LSD and psychedelic drugs, drugs that were entirely legal just a few years before the iconic Summer of Love. As the hippie era of psychedelic cinema ended, no film revealed the truth about LSD and how it triggered one of the greatest leaps in consciousness since the invention of film itself. It would have to wait another half century, when once classified documents and brave researchers and writers were finally able to tell the true tale of LSD. It's an ever-evolving one as new scientific breakthroughs are occurring even now in the realms of psychedelic medicine. But as far as truth serums and the CIA's quest to find one, they did, in something called the Devil's Breath—Scopolamine.

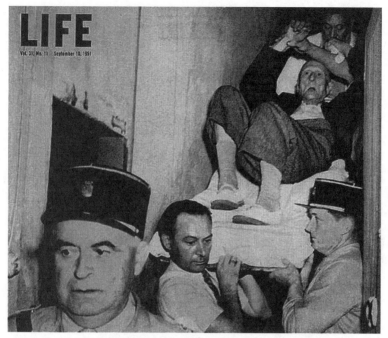

The Pont-Saint-Esprit acid attack (*Life*)

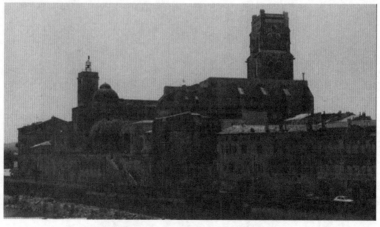

Pont-Saint-Esprit (*Wiki Commons*)

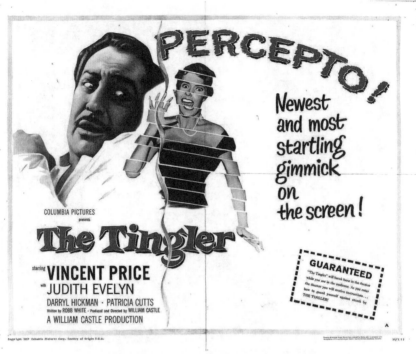

The Tingler, 1959 (Colombia Pictures)

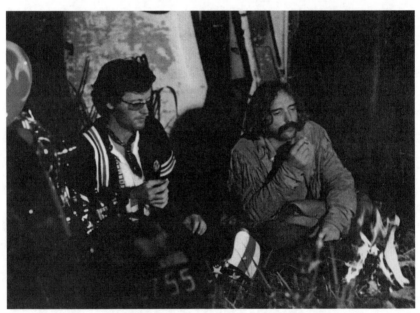

Peter Fonda and Dennis Hopper in *Easy Rider* (*The Red List*)

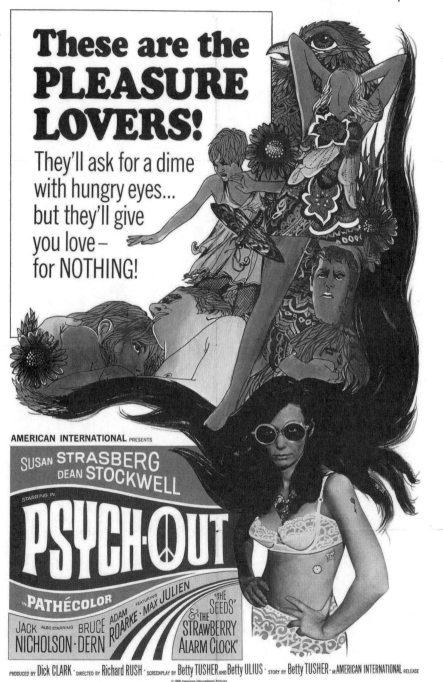

Psych-Out, 1968 (American International Pictures)

Chapter Nine

Scopolamine:
The CIA's Real Truth Serum

America is not so much a nightmare as a non-dream.
The American non-dream is precisely a move to wipe
the dream out of existence. The dream is a spontaneous
happening and therefore dangerous to a control system
set up by the non-dreamers.
—William S. Burroughs

Scopolamine was first used along with morphine and chloroform in the early 1900s by physicians wishing to induce a state of "twilight sleep" during childbirth. A constituent of henbane, scopolamine produced sedation, confusion and disorientation, sometimes even amnesia for events experienced during intoxication. Despite this, physicians noted that women in twilight sleep answered questions accurately and candidly, seemingly unable to lie. In 1922, Robert House, a Dallas obstetrician, employed scopolamine in the interrogation of two suspected criminals, who both denied the charges on which they were held, and upon trial, both were found not guilty. Excited at this success, House concluded that a patient under the influence of scopolamine "cannot create a lie ...and there is no power to think or reason"[1] and thus the idea of a truth drug was born. House published 11 articles about scopolamine in the years 1921-1929, an eight-year scientific crusade that saw the father of the truth serum go largely unnoticed in the public eye. Policemen of the time liked to use the drug as an interrogation tool, but the number of undesirable side effects associated with scopolamine when not administered in the correct dosage disqualified it as a reliable truth drug. Among the worst side effects are hallucinations, somnolence, and physiological attacks like headaches, rapid heart rates, and blurred vision, which distract the subject from the purpose of the interview. Furthermore, the extreme case of dry mouth brought on by the drug is hardly conducive to talkative chatter. And although it was ditched early by police as an interrogation device, leave it to the CIA to once again show everyone how it's done.

Scopolamine, otherwise known as Devil's Breath, is derived from the seeds of the Borrachero tree, part of the 'nightshade' tree family that includes henbane and Angel's Trumpet, all of which figure into the mixture of the drug, a powerful concoction that causes memory loss by limiting or stifling the function of the acetylcholine neurotransmitter. Acetylcholine is located within the part of the brain that records your memories onto a perpetual stream of newly formed brain cells. In the drug world, scopolamine is classified as an anticholinergic, and described as a deliriant able to produce hallucinations that leave the user in a vulnerable state without free will. Eventually in their quest for a "truth serum" the CIA stumbled upon scopolamine in the early 50s and began their own experiments and research into the drug. Yhe drug wasn't a leap into the next dimension as LSD provided, but a divisive compound that seemed more likely to create a Manchurian candidate, easy to control. If the CIA handlers were to keep a subject strung out on scopolamine for an extended period of time, they would have the perfect operative with no behavioral filters of morality or ethics, like a robot without reason that suffers zero mental side effects. But what's the use of a truth serum that only creates an army of zombies?

More tests were needed and other agencies got involved, as NASA discovered that scopolamine counters the effects of motion sickness, and the NSA used it illegally for decades on their own agents. Eventually the dirty little secret that scopolamine was the mind control drug of choice and ultimate truth serum began to leak out in the late 2010s. In high doses, the drug can make the victim black out and do whatever they are told for a window of six hours, with no memory of the darkened period. One possible scenario you could exploit with a Manchurian candidate under the influence of scopolamine would be that of a "lone nut" shooter who is backed up by a team of black ops commandos that go in and shoot up a movie theater or something. This event happened in Colorado when supposed shooter James Holmes, the son of a CIA biochemical expert, shot up the cinema during the premiere of the Batman flick *The Dark Knight Rises*. Was the shooter under the influence of scopolamine during the incident?

Scopolamine in its purest form can be still found in Colombia where dealers of the potion say they can blow it into the face of a victim and put them under their control. It's commonly used by thieves and scammers in South American countries to render victims helpless while they steal all their money and valuables. The drug might have been used on John P. Wheeler III, an Illuminati insider and former biological weapons contractor with the Bush family crime syndicate. By the time of his mysterious and still unsolved death, scopolamine was the drug of choice for intelligence agencies looking to induce zombie-like states in their victims, who were then able to follow any orders given to them. Using it for various purposes, such as a truth serum, to create a patsy, or for blackmail by getting the victim to engage in blackmailable activities that they would have never otherwise engaged in, scopolamine was the breakthrough spy drug the CIA had been looking for since the 1940s. Based on the eyewitness reports specifically mentioning that Wheeler had red eyes, and exhibited the other hallmarks of being under the influence of the drug, it's safe to say that scopolamine played a major part in his death. Wheeler was seen disoriented, in a delirious state, wandering around downtown Wilmington, Delaware after apparently being robbed:

Events surrounding the murder of John P. Wheeler III, who most recently worked part-time for defense contractor Mitre Corporation on cyber defense topics, read like a Tom Clancy novel. The 66-year-old worked for three Republican administrations, was special assistant to the Secretary of the Air Force, served in the office of the Secretary of Defense, and penned a manual on the effectiveness of biological and chemical weapons, which urged US forces to show restraint. The day after Christmas—five days before his body was found as it was being dumped from a trash truck

155

into the Cherry Island Landfill in Wilmington—Wheeler sent longtime friend Richard Radez an email expressing concern that the US wasn't sufficiently prepared for "cyber warfare," according to The Associated Press. "This was something that had preoccupied him over the last couple of years," Radez told the news organization. Wheeler's focus on computer warfare, and his ties to Mitre, have already attracted conspiracy theories involving the military industrial complex, but there are plenty of other intriguing details that don't immediately fit into such a plot. Among them are revelations that Wheeler was seen on December 29 and 30 in a "confused and disoriented" state in downtown Wilmington. During that last appearance, which occurred some 14 hours before his body was discovered, he was wandering inside an office building a few blocks from an attorney who was handling a contentious lawsuit Wheeler filed to stop neighbors from building a home near his. He refused help from several people who approached him. A day earlier, he approached a parking garage attendant "wearing a black suit with no tie and only one shoe," according to the AP report. He carried the missing shoe in his hand and wore no overcoat, despite the frigid temperature. He told the attendant he had been robbed of his briefcase and said repeatedly he wasn't drunk. To further the intrigue, Delaware police have reportedly found evidence that Wheeler may have been involved in an attempted arson on the same neighbors he was suing. The attempted arson on December 28 came after someone tossed several smoke bombs used for rodent control into the neighbors' house, scorching the floors. What's more, the AP has reported that yellow police evidence tape was seen surrounding two wooden chairs in Wheeler's kitchen, where several wooden floorboards were missing, even though Delaware police have said the victim's home is not considered a crime scene. A neighbor, according to Examiner.com, said Wheeler's television blared continuously in the days preceding his death. Those details, combined with the fact that someone went to considerable effort to hide Wheeler's body in a trash dumpster in nearby Newark, Delaware, would suggest the homicide wasn't a random mugging.[2]

Russian intelligence uses scopolamine under the codename SP-11, usually in the form of candy given to unwilling victims. This was the case in 1955, when Lisa Stein, an interviewer with RIAS, the American propaganda radio station in West Germany, was fed candy containing scopolamine:

> It was intended that Frau Stein would become ill and would be abducted. The plan was that the agent —someone whom Frau Stein trusted and with whom she was meeting in a West Berlin café —would offer the poisoned candy toward the end of the meeting. The lady was expected to become ill while walking from the cafe to her nearby residence. On becoming unconscious, she was to be picked up by a waiting car which would appear to be passing by chance. The plot was not carried to fruition, however, because Frau Stein did not become ill until she was near her apartment, at which point neighbors came to her aid and she was moved to a hospital. She was severely ill for 48 hours, after which an antidote was found. (Unclassified, from the testimony of Theodor Hans, formerly with U.S. Military Intelligence, Germany, September 21, 1960, before a Congressional investigating committee.)[3]

Ted Gunderson, a retired FBI agent, interviewed Gene "Chip" Tatum, a former CIA black ops assassin and Illuminati insider for a provocative piece of video journalism known on Youtube as *Presidential Secrets*. Chip Tatum illustrates how the zombie drug, when used properly, was a favorite of intelligence agencies, as a truth serum and drug that made people willing to do whatever they were told. Chip was involved in Operation Red Rock, Task Force 160 and OSG2, all topsecret programs that did the dirty work of covert CIA killing sprees and narcotrafficking with a little scopolamine sprinkled in for kidnaps and assassinations. Illuminati historian Fritz Springmeier documented Chip's views on scopolamine being the key to creating a totally undetectable mind controlled slave by combing through 12 hours of Ted Gundersson's interview transcripts:

> Well, you know, it can be used in many manners. You can put it in tobacco. You can put it in a soda. You can put it in a punch-bowl. It's odorless and tasteless. The results of the drug are a complete-control situation. We—it's nicknamed "borodanga" (sp?), but it actually comes from the nightshade family of a flowering shrub that is pretty well found in Central and South America. Depending on the member of the family that you use, your results will be a little different. We used a particular nightshade bulb for the—for our voodoo drug, as we called it, but a person can be under the control of the voodoo drug, Ted, and you can tell them to go to the bank and withdraw all their funds from the bank, and they'll go do it. The bank-teller can't tell that they're under any influence of any drug. They'll return it to you, and the following day, when they go to the bank, or two days later, when they go to the bank, to get their money out, they won't remember that they withdrew it all and gave it to you. Once we had a person on a derivative of scopolamine, escopolaminia (sp?), we didn't need anything else. We could control them for up to three weeks, and, during that three weeks, we could actually alter their personality, so, you know, there was no real requirement for shock—unless, for some reason, there were some discipline problems, or body—you know, the body-size required too much of the drug to take effect. But that was rarely the case. You know, we lost a few people, from overdoses, but that's about it.[4]

When properly administered scopolamine causes absolute obedience without being observable by others, and more importantly, the target won't recall any of the events that occurred during the period they were under the drug's spell. Shortly after shooting the interview, Chip suddenly disappeared in the winter of 1998; it's rumored that his tortured body washed up on a beach in Panama a decade later. In the end, LSD would be pushed aside as a failed truth serum that inadvertently spawned the rise of the hippies, while scopolamine, the agency's greatest black arts gift, would go largely unnoticed or unmentioned except for hipster hit pieces on *Vice*. But the psychedelic renaissance failed to go quietly into the night, as a new breed of doctors, scientists and explorers continued to blaze new paths on the never-ending quest to understand the psychedelic liquid conspiracy, finding potential hope for medical and mental health breakthroughs thanks to the magic mushrooms found at the end of a technicolor rainbow.

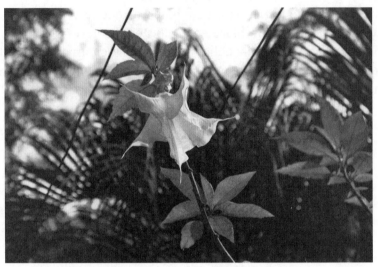

The Scopolamine Flower *(Business Insider)*

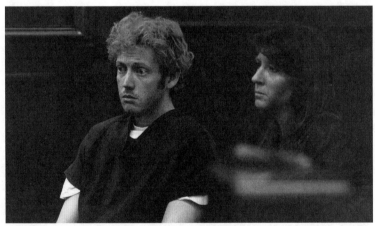

James Holmes, the Scopolamine Manchurian Candidate? *(AP)*

Chapter Ten

The Magic Mushrooms at the End of the Rainbow

Thousands of years before Christianity, secret cults arose which worshipped the sacred mushroom—the Amanita Muscaria—which, for various reasons (including its shape and power as a drug) came to be regarded as a symbol of God on earth. When the secrets of the cult had to be written down, it was done in the form of codes hidden in folk tales. This is the basic origin of the stories in the New Testament. They are a literary device to spread the rites and rules of mushroom worship to the faithful.
—John Allegro, *The Sacred Mushroom and the Cross*

It was a cloudy, thunder-filled day when I first discovered the magic mushrooms at the end of the rainbow. I was with my cousin and his father, and we were exploring the gulley behind a row of run-down houses on the city's inglorious east side. In the 1990s, Tacoma was notorious for being a blue-collar hellhole, full of tweekers, gangbangers and overall tough times. It had been years since my uncle was actively involved in my cousin's life; he ditched the family while everyone was still in middle school, opting to be a beach bum far away in Hawaii instead. In his absence, my aunt sunk into a meth habit as the family moved into the projects. For my cousin jail would replace school, and eventually any promise that once existed for a brighter future began its slow fade-out. But on that particular day, the light raindrops of the evening mists didn't bother us at all as we searched patches of grass for a certain blue-ringed mushroom. Known locally as blue ringers, these magic mushrooms are native to the Pacific Northwest and usually pop up during the fall season near Halloween. Originally found growing on the University of Washington campus, they went unnoticed for god knows how long until being plucked by curious mycologist Daniel Stuntz, who determined them to be in the psychedelic class. *Psilocybe stuntzii*, named after its discoverer, is a psilocybin mushroom of the Hymenogastraceae family, having psilocybin and psilocin as main active compounds, and is similar to the more popular *Psilocybe semilanceata* (liberty caps).

"Here we go…got'em," my uncle proclaimed as he plucked a few shrooms and lifted them high to inspect them up close. Drops of rain gliding from his black dangling curls, he drew us in to inspect the properties of the magical mushroom, pointing out the blue rings native to each one. He dropped them into an empty Doritos bag and, now knowing what to look, for we spread out hunting for blue-ringed mushrooms. By the time my Doritos bag was full, I was waved over by my uncle and my cousin, and the three of us proceeded to march back home with bags full of psychedelic goodies. After the shrooms had been cleaned and dried, they sat in a huge bowl on the kitchen table. When the pizza arrived it was quickly covered with the magical caps and devoured by the ravenous appetites of psychedelic rookies. It might have been one cap too many, but for my third eye it was love at first sight. It really started to kick in about halfway through that night's episode of *WCW Monday Nitro*, and became an ongoing freight train of rainbows that glistened in the valleys of the popcorn ceiling I was staring at while trying to fall asleep. It might have worn off sometime after the Prince Naseem Hamed blowout of Steve Robinson the next afternoon, but since there was still a huge bowl of mushrooms sitting on the kitchen table, I and everyone else kept shoving them into our mouths. The taste was horrendous, and to this day I can't stand eating mushrooms unless they are of the magical kind. The best way to enjoy them is by way of tea; this makes it far easier—to drink as a sweet delight rather than a quick swallowing of tasteless disgust. Unlike acid, I've never had a bad trip on shrooms, the trip seems to be far more controllable and less intense if administered in the proper dose. The tracers and highlighting of colors and the opening of senses make shrooms great for both the visual and musical arts; movies like *Alien* and *Apocalypse Now* are greatly enhanced by the psilocybin mushroom experience.

Although the CIA did numerous tests with magic mushrooms, they quickly determined they were of no threat or real use to the agency, but still realized they were mind opening enough not to let *you* have them. The magic mushroom fell into the illegal drugs category along with the rest of the psychedelics. But modern day tests of the funky fungi have uncovered the enzymatic pathways that allow mushrooms to create psilocybin, that when converted by the body into the molecule psilocin, produces the groovy vibes and hallucinogenic effects that we're all used to. Although CIA scientists have known the chemical structure of psilocybin since the 50s, the biochemcial pathways that allow shrooms to make the psychedelic compound have been a mystery until now. Researchers at Friedrich Schiller University in Jena, Germany have isolated the four enzymes used to make psilocybin in magic mushrooms and created the first enzymatic synthesis of psilocybin, a groundbreaking step towards commercializing the compound for mass production. For the study, published in the German science journal *Angewandte Chemie*, researchers sequenced the genomes of two different species of magic mushroom: Psilocybe cubensis and Psilocybe cyanescens. *Gizmodo's* George Dvorksy explains how the genome sequencing process works:

> It starts with a special kind of tryptophan molecule, with an extra oxygen and hydrogen stuck on, like an anglerfish with a big head and a tail and an extra piece hanging off like the headlight. An enzyme the researchers named PsiD first strips a carbon dioxide molecule off of the tail. Then, an enzyme they called PsiK phosphorylates it, meaning it replaces the headlight's oxygen with a special setup of phosphorus with some oxygen attached. A final enzyme, called PsiM, works to replace two hydrogen atoms on the tail with methyl groups, or carbon atoms with three hydrogens attached.[1]

After figuring out how mushrooms make psilocybin, researchers genetically modified E. coli bacteria that then synthetically produced the enzymes involved in the psilocybin compound's production, laying the foundation for developing a fermentation process of the powerful psychedelic fungus, which has a fascinating history and pharmacology. Although psilocybin has long been abandoned and disregarded by the scientific community, thanks to it being an illegal drug, recent studies have shown that the compound can be helpful in treating a host of psychological conditions. Psilocybin has been shown to reduce anxiety in patients with life-threatening cancers, alleviate symptoms of depression, and even help people kick alcohol and nicotine habits. But since psilocybin is still a controlled substance in America, it might be decades more before it is accepted by the mainstream as a medical treatment. But the new studies are a promising step in unlocking the healing powers of the funky mushroom, as researchers involved in the trials say the results were remarkable. Volunteers that signed up for the psychedelic tests claimed to have had "profoundly meaningful and spiritual experiences"[2] which ended their depression and made them rethink life. The results of the research published in the *Journal of Psychopharmacology,* together with commentaries from leading scientists in the fields of psychiatry and palliative care, all back further scientific studies of the magic mushroom. But do they back its legalization?

The effects of magic mushrooms have been of interest to psychiatry since the 1950s, but the classification of all psychedelics in America as Schedule I drugs after the rise of the hippie counterculture, has made the legal and financial obstacles to running the trials almost impossible to overcome, leaving us at a crossroads of what to do with this monumental scientific breakthrough. "I think it is a big deal both in terms of the findings and in terms of the history and what it represents. It was part of psychiatry and vanished and now it's been brought back,"[3] said Dr. Stephen Ross, director of addiction psychiatry at NYU Langone Medical Center and lead investigator of one of the studies tested there. Almost half of newly diagnosed cancer patients suffer depression and suicidal thoughts; these vibes are only negatively enhanced when prescribed the usual anti-depression medications, however when replaced with psilocybin there's an immediate reduction in depression and anxiety. Professor Roland Griffiths, of the departments of psychiatry and neuroscience, who led the study at Johns Hopkins University school of medicine, described the results as nothing short of remarkable. "I am bred as a skeptic. I was skeptical at the outset that this drug could produce long-lasting changes," said the professor. But he noted that people "facing the deepest existential questions that humans can encounter—what is the nature of life and death, the meaning of life... In spite of their unique vulnerability and the mood disruption that the illness and contemplation of their death has prompted, these participants have the same kind of experiences, that are deeply meaningful, spiritually significant and producing enduring positive changes in life and mood and behavior." Patients described the experiences as "re-organizational" and "mystical," using unscientific terms at a loss to explain how psilocybin activates a sub-type of ancient serotonin receptor in the brain. A scientist quoted in The Smithsonian Magazine article about this research said:

Our brains are hard-wired to have these kinds of experiences—these alterations of consciousness. We have endogenous chemicals in our brain. We have a little system that, when you tickle it, it produces these altered states that have been described as spiritual states, mystical states in different religious branches. They are defined by a sense of oneness—people feel that their separation between the personal ego and the outside world is sort of dissolved and they feel that they are part of some continuous energy or consciousness in the universe. Patients can feel sort of transported to a different dimension of reality, sort of like a waking dream.[4]

Perhaps it's time to step back into the 1950s and 1960s and start to take psychedelic treatments in psychiatry and oncology seriously, as we did then. Most participants in the new studies of psilocybin agree that we're in an exciting new phase of psychedelic psychopharmacology that should be encouraged not encumbered. The studies were funded by the Heffter Research Institute whose medical director George Greer concluded, "These findings, the most profound to date in the medical use of psilocybin, indicate it could be more effective at treating serious psychiatric diseases than traditional pharmaceutical approaches, and without having to take a medication every day."⁵ Yes indeed. But the hippie mystic, a staple of American youth culture for half a century, found across the nation's college campuses and identifiable by their Dead Head philosophies on the cosmic benefits of mushrooms and other hallucinogenic substances are still around. Their vibe's still threatened by "the man" looking to throw them into the prison industrial complex slave mill, just for some gnarly tasting shrooms that grow in the wild.

The countercultural magic mushroom craze all started with a humble Mazateca shaman from Huatla de Jiménez by the name of María Sabina, who had been performing psychedelic healing rituals called veladas since her childhood. Banking executive R. Gordon Wasson tracked María Sabina down after reading ancient Spanish codexes that spoke of Aztec magic mushroom rituals. Wasson made his way to Huatla de Jiménez, where he met María Sabina who performed the velada ritual on the curious gringo, who ended up returning eight more times. He even brought with him *Life* magazine, Timothy Leary and of course the CIA, who experimented with psilocybin during their infamous MK-ULTRA mind control experiments. Huatla de Jiménez became a tourist destination for adventurous hipster mushroom-munching mystics. María Sabina was shunned by her community for commercializing their traditions and died in poverty, but not before turning on the likes of Bob Dylan and John Lennon.

The ancient Mayan codexes weren't the only ancient manuscripts that talked about magic mushrooms. The Bible spoke about the sacred "manna" that the Israelites ate while wandering around in the desert. The Bible describes manna as a small round edible object that appeared after dew had fallen on the ground. If the manna was exposed for too long in the Sun, it would get worms and stink worse than it tastes. Exodus 16:14-20: And when the dew that lay was gone up, behold, upon the face of the wilderness there lay a small round thing, as small as the hoar frost on the ground...some of them left of it till the morning, and it bred worms, and stank.⁶

Was this small, round, edible object—which when left in the Sun rots, breeds worms, and stinks—none other than the magic mushroom? James Arthur, once the world's foremost ethnomycologist writes in *Mushrooms and Mankind*:

> Manna was thought of as being produced miraculously (IE: birth without seed). This is a perfect botanical description of a mushroom. Birth without seed (miraculous) is due to spores being microscopic and not visible to the naked eye. Jesus describes the Mannas in detail in the book of John. In this story Jesus attempts to make clear; of manna, there are two different ones/kinds. He describes the manna that he is giving the disciples (last supper) as the Manna that bestows immortality. His statement, unless you have eaten his flesh/body (Soma/Manna), and drink of his blood (Soma Juice), you have no life in you, takes on a whole new meaning in light of this discovery. The Manna is directly associated with the fruit of the Tree of Life in the 2nd chapter of the book of Revelation. It is the reward for those who overcome (the lies of the world). The 'Fruit of the Tree', the 'Hidden Manna' and the 'Small White Stone' are spoken of separately, but in the same context. All of these are symbols for the Amanita muscaria.[7]

The church, its priests and pastors have all denied that manna was a magic mushroom and insist instead that it represents a bread from heaven, despite having a difficult time refuting its description as a small, round dew-covered thing found in the wilderness as described in the Bible. Also, bread, unless covered in ergot doesn't contain any of the mystical properties bestowed upon it like the magic mushroom does. James Arthur continues:

> The concept of the literal ingestion of the body of God is highly downplayed by religious scholars of today. The body (soma) being a fleshy Mushroom is much more palatable than trying to stomach cannibalism or the transformation of ordinary substances. Many questions should be asked about this cosmopolitan idea of the 'Sacramental Substance'. Unfortunately, the religious experts shun the notion, insisting that the entire idea is nothing more than symbolic. A symbol points at something

else, not usually at another symbology. The Catholic church, in the early 1100's, decided to have the final word on this subject by establishing (under Emperor/Pope Innocent III) the 'Doctrine of Trans-Substantiation'. This is whereby, the Priests, by their assumed holy power, claim to be able to say some magical words, and turn ordinary bread into the literal 'Body of God'. This event is one of the biggest evil deceptions of all time, is an undermining of the basic esoteric aspects of the religion, and is, arguably, the most horrible and damning event to ever happen to Christendom, and as such the entire human race. Jesus clearly describes the Manna that he calls his body in the book of John. Repeatedly describing the 'Thing/Manna' as a substance hidden from the world, but revealed to his disciples. Understanding the last supper story becomes as simplistic as it gets, if you know how to decipher the event. Adamantly; Jesus says, 'Take and eat, This is my Body.' This is saying pretty clearly that the eating and drinking is physical. My body is flesh indeed, and my blood is drink indeed, and the added statement that when you eat, it is inside of you leaves little room for debate that this is a substance, not a phantom symbol alone. For those who choose to debate this I ask that they show me their substance because according to Jesus' words unless you eat and drink of 'It' you have no life in you. By the way, do I really need to mention that this is not some strange reference to Cannibalism? I sure hope not, if you still think this, read on. Somewhere, some of this must convince you that he is not saying to take a bite out of his arm, or any other piece of his actual anatomy... In my opinion, the magical act of 'Trans-Substantiation' has no merit. The statement that Jesus makes 'Unless you eat and drink you have no life in you' would seem to condemn the replacement of whatever the real thing is with a placebo (substitute).[8]

John Allegro, *Dead Sea Scrolls* scholar and respected archaeologist, had his career ruined after publishing *The Sacred Mushroom and the Cross* in 1970, a twenty-year study of Semitic and proto-Semitic languages alluding to fertility cults using the sacred mushroom, Amanita muscaria, as a gateway to divine understanding. Allegro discovered that this sacred psychedelic magic mushroom was at the root of many religions, including early Christianity, but the critics and the public couldn't get past the initial shockwaves caused after the book's release. The magic mushroom cloud of Allegro's thesis spread more derision than enlightenment, and *The Sacred Mushroom and the Cross*, a universally vilified book, fell out of print and out of mind for almost 40 years. But since then, new linguistic and non-linguistic evidence has come to light in support of many of Allegro's theories, including Russian linguist Vladimir Nikolaevic Toporov's 1985 paper "On the Semiotics of Mythological Conceptions about Mushrooms," as well as Jan Irvin's *The Holy Mushroom: Evidence of Mushrooms in Judeo-Christianity*. The 16th century Christian text *The Epistle to the Renegade Bishops* explicitly discusses "the holy mushroom."

The sacred magic mushroom might soon be made available to at least one section of the public soon after the time this book hits the shelves. In the state of Californian, citizens will get the chance to vote on "Magic Mushroom Legalization"[9] in 2018, voting on whether to decriminalize the use of hallucinogenic mushrooms under a newly proposed ballot measure which was filed with the state Attorney General's office in 2017. The bill would exempt people ages 21 and over from criminal penalties for using, possessing, selling, transporting or cultivating psilocybin, a hallucinogenic compound found in certain mushroom species. With marijuana already legalized in California, hopefully it's just a matter of time before psilocybin legalization is also introduced to the Sunshine State. This would be a logical and beneficial thing, considering that recent studies have shown that psilocybin compounds can provide benefits to cancer patients as well as treat other psychological ailments. A recent global survey also revealed that magic mushrooms are the most fun and safest of all recreational drugs, and are more prone to leading users through the doors of perception, rather than the doors of the emergency room.

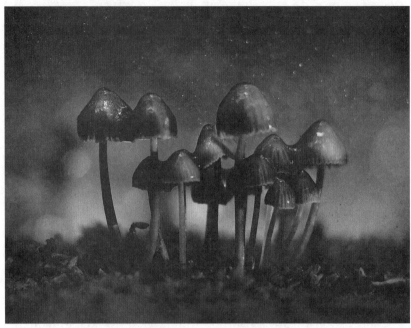

Magic mushrooms could be among safest drugs, new survey finds (*Business Insider*)

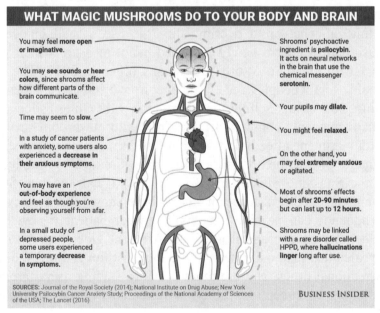

WHAT MAGIC MUSHROOMS DO TO YOUR BODY AND BRAIN

You may feel **more open or imaginative.**

You may **see sounds or hear colors,** since shrooms affect how different parts of the brain communicate.

Time may seem to **slow.**

In a study of cancer patients with anxiety, some users also experienced a **decrease in their anxious symptoms.**

You may have an **out-of-body experience** and feel as though you're observing yourself from afar.

In a small study of depressed people, some users experienced a temporary **decrease in symptoms.**

Shrooms' psychoactive ingredient is **psilocybin.** It acts on neural networks in the brain that use the chemical messenger **serotonin.**

Your pupils may **dilate.**

You might feel **relaxed.**

On the other hand, you may feel **extremely anxious** or agitated.

Most of shrooms' effects begin after **20-90 minutes** but can last up to **12 hours.**

Shrooms may be linked with a rare disorder called HPPD, where **hallucinations linger** long after use.

SOURCES: Journal of the Royal Society (2014); National Institute on Drug Abuse; New York University Psilocybin Cancer Anxiety Study; Proceedings of the National Academy of Sciences of the USA; The Lancet (2016)

BUSINESS INSIDER

What Magic Mushrooms do to your body and brain (*Business Insider*)

170

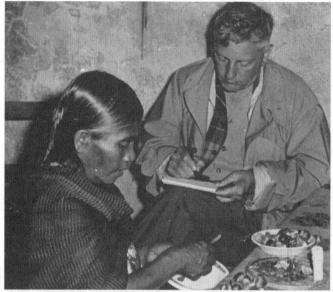

Maria Sabina, the Mazatec curandera who introduced R. Gordon
Wasson to magic mushrooms (*Pinterest*)

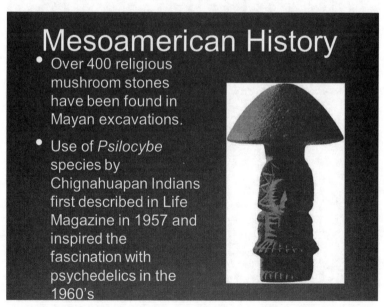

Mesoamerican History

- Over 400 religious mushroom stones have been found in Mayan excavations.

- Use of *Psilocybe* species by Chignahuapan Indians first described in Life Magazine in 1957 and inspired the fascination with psychedelics in the 1960's

Magic Mushrooms in Mesoamerican history *(Pinterest)*

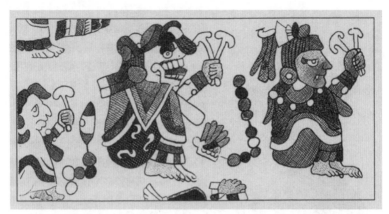

Mayan Deities with magic mushrooms (*The Herb Museum*)

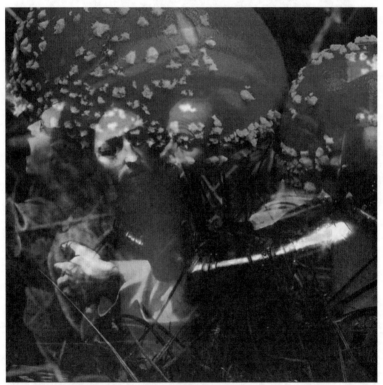

John Allegro's The Sacred Mushroom and the Cross: Was Jesus
actually a "magic mushroom"? (*Night Flight*)

Chapter Eleven

Big Pharma's War on Psychedelics

"But I don't want to go among mad people," Alice remarked.
"Oh, you can't help that," said the Cat, "we're all mad here. I'm
mad. You're mad."
"How do you know I'm mad?" said Alice.
"You must be," said the Cat, "or you wouldn't have come here."
—Lewis Carroll, *Alice in Wonderland*

Unfortunately, the war on drugs endlessly marches on. Will psychedelic drug research survive? Currently, psychedelic research is undergoing a renaissance, but the promising field may be in danger thanks to outdated neocon relic Jeff Sessions, a man hellbent on restoring the good ol' days of throwing everyone in jail for "drugs." After the 1970s Controlled Substance Act lamely criminalized all psychedelics, there was a long period of silence in American psychedelic research that persisted until 2002, when over twenty studies were approved. The landmark research on MDMA-assisted therapy for veterans suffering from PTSD came from one of these studies, and for the first time since the CIA was running amok with aerosol cans of LSD, science was beginning to see the light in regard to the healing powers of psychedelics. But even though President Donald Trump ran on a platform that promised not to harass states with legalized medical and recreational marijuana, Sessions has become fixated with linking marijuana to the rise of opium abuse and has been actively seeking to shut down the legal marijuana industry in the United States. This infighting doesn't bode well as far as psychedelics are concerned, considering they are viewed as far more dangerous than pot, at least in the eyes of Sessions and the DEA. The FDA also calls the shots far more than any president ever could, maintaining the medical monopoly that has seen profits soar over 250% in the last decade.[1]

Both the FDA and DEA benefit greatly from the phony war on drugs. The DEA is overseen by the Department of Justice (DOJ) which is under the supervision of Jeff Sessions, who has already been caught asking Congress to allow him to prosecute marijuana cases in states that have legalized medical and recreational marijuana. No word yet on what the agency plans on doing with the psychedelic agenda, but increased law enforcement action from the DOJ concerning marijuana is probably enough to scare scientists away from any further psychedelic research. However, Rick Doblin, executive director of psychedelic research nonprofit MAPS, a leading funder of psychedelic research, feels very optimistic about the future of psychedelics, saying, "One of the Trump administration's main things is lower regulation. They're pro business and pro making it easier for Big Pharma to get drugs through the FDA. And that benefits us."[2] But the FDA isn't boss hog as far as influential agencies goes; in order to conduct psychedelic research a DEA license is required. To combat this, deregulation is needed, but psychedelics remain Schedule I drugs and are categorized among a class of substances purported to have no medical benefits and high risk of abuse. Schedule I drug offenses also bring the harshest penalties for possession and recreational use, leading to years in prison. Literally the most dangerous thing about psychedelics is getting caught with them!

Any clinical or medical use of psychedelics in America must go through a rigorous DEA licensing and FDA approval process, that is costly, time consuming and mostly futile. Psychedelic research chemist and pharmacologist David Nichols, president of the Heffter Research Institute, which has funded 12 FDA-approved clinical psychedelic studies since the late 90s, doesn't believe that Congress will change the current drug laws anytime soon. "We're just a flea on the back of this dog,"[3] Nichols says in regards to the golden goose that is the drug industry, seeing no hope of allowing any natural psychedelia found in nature to ever compete against the many-headed man-made hydras of the medical and deep state cartels. Despite having to fight Sessions over the future of drugs, Trump's FDA commissioner Scott Gottlieb has made "deregulation" one of his key talking points, endorsing cuts in the regulatory processes in favor of quick drug approvals—although he hasn't specifically addressed the areas of psychedelic research. Marijuana isn't a psychedelic, yet it's subject to even stricter research regulations despite being legal in eight states and permitted for medical use in 30. The DOJ's renewed hardline stance on marijuana is likely to kill any further research on "illegal" drugs, and since psychedelics aren't legal anywhere, getting approval for drugs like psilocybin will likely decline. Though researchers know more than ever about psychedelic drugs, including their promising potential uses—none of that positive research has translated over to law enforcement policy, where established drug laws target people of color and low-income communities, with mandatory incarceration for drug possession. With Sessions unwilling to consider research suggesting medical marijuana actually helps some people, it's unlikely he'll push for any kind of reform for psychedelics, either. And this ancient line of thinking does more harm than good, improving the prison industrial complex which creates a form of slave labor. This slave labor at 10 cents an hour in effect keeps the wages low in the outside world, as businesses struggle to keep up financially with the cheap prison labor workforce. If you don't think the whole war on drugs is a scam, ask yourself this—why is 80% of the prison population only there on drug charges? If these so-called "drugs" were legal, there wouldn't be such a large prison population! You're being sentenced to a life of slave labor for a mere life choice, and valuable medical and scientific research is being prevented thanks to these "drugs" that were written on a "drugs are bad m'kay" list in the 1970s.

But the psychedelic renaissance marches on with MDMA, a drug more commonly found on dance floors in Ibiza, and known as Molly or ecstasy. More than ten prestigious universities partnered with the psilocybin-focused Heffter Research Institute to study the compound for smoking cessation, alcoholism, terminal-cancer anxiety and PTSD to surprising positive results:

> Since 2000, the Multidisciplinary Association for Psychedelic Studies (MAPS), a nonprofit based in Santa Cruz, California, has been funding clinical trials of MDMA

for subjects with PTSD, mostly veterans, but also police, firefighters and civilians. In November, the FDA approved large-scale Phase III clinical trials—the last phase before potential medicalization—of MDMA for PTSD treatment. MAPS, which has committed $25 million to achieving that medicalization by 2021, also supports or runs research with ayahuasca (a concoction of Amazonian plants), LSD, medical marijuana and ibogaine, the pharmaceutical extract of the psychoactive African shrub iboga. The organization is additionally funding a study of MDMA for treating social anxiety in autistic adults, currently underway at UCLA Medical Center. Another study, using MDMA to treat anxiety in patients with life-threatening illnesses, has concluded.[4]

MDMA-assisted psychotherapy and PTSD studies funded by MAPS, have been met with an overarching negative political climate, but the biggest challenge for the researchers isn't federal regulation—it's fundraising. Trump's proposed budget for 2018 has a 16.2 percent cut for The U.S. Department of Health and Human Services (HHS). Psychedelic research has never received government grants from HHS departments, so no noticeable loss there, but if more scientists are forced to find private funding to continue working, psychedelics might slide to the bottom of the list for potential donors. This is a huge setback, since the recent surge in compelling clinical data should encourage HHS to finally lend financial support to psychedelic research. Clinical studies are expensive some costing over a million dollars, but years of lobbying and laboratory research on the medical uses of MDMA, has forced the FDA to move forward with studies of the drug after announcing that MAPS made a clinical breakthrough with MDMA used as a treatment for PTSD. Ecstasy, the popular recreational drug, whose main ingredient is MDMA has been shown to unlock far more than just fly dance moves, providing significant relief for sufferers of PTSD in clinical use trials conducted over the past several years. The FDA granted MAPS, which has been championing MDMA research for 30 years, a Breakthrough Therapy Designation, indicating the agency believes the treatment rivals the current available medications for PTSD. MAPS has also reached an agreement with the FDA under the Special Protocol Assessment Process for the design of two future Phase III trials for MDMA-assisted psychotherapy for patients with PTSD. "Reaching agreement with [the] FDA on the design of our Phase 3 program and having the ability to work closely with the agency has been a major priority for our team. Our Phase 2 data was extremely promising with a large effect size, and we are ready to move forward quickly. With breakthrough designation, we can now move even more efficiently through the development process in collaboration with the FDA to complete Phase 3."[5] said Amy Emerson, Executive Director of the MAPS Public Benefit Corporation. Rick Doblin, Founder and Executive Director of MAPS, commented, "For the first time ever, psychedelic-assisted psychotherapy will be evaluated in Phase 3 trials for possible prescription use, with MDMA-assisted psychotherapy for PTSD leading the way ...Now that we have agreement with FDA, we are ready to start negotiations with the European Medicines Agency."[6]

Phase II trials completed by MAPS saw 61% of its participants no longer qualify for PTSD aid two months after they underwent three sessions of MDMA-assisted psychotherapy. The placebo-controlled Phase III trials of MDMA-assisted psychotherapy with groups of 200 to 300 participants with PTSD aged 18 and over will take place at monitored sites in America, Canada, and Israel in the spring of 2018 if MAPS can obtain the estimated $25 million needed to conduct the project. David Nutt, an influential neuropsychopharmacologist at Imperial College London, has been waiting a long time for some mainstream acceptance of MDMA. "This is not a big scientific step ...It's been obvious for 40 years that these drugs are medicines. But it's a huge step in acceptance,"[7] he told *Science*. Far from the neon dancefloors where you'll usually find MDMA is a different psychedelic wonder that grows in the emerald rain forests of South America.

Ayahuasca, a powerful hallucinogenic vine long revered by Amazonian shaman's as a tool for peering deep into the soul, is going under the microscope as neuroscientists in Aerica begin studying the sacred psychedelic. The ritual treatment of drinking a well-stewed tea containing ayahuasca has drawn interest from foreign visitors wishing to partake in the ceremonies commonly held in the mountains of Peru. Made famous by the writings of Graham Hancock and popularized even more by the Joe Rogan podcast, the mystical "vine of souls," as it is called in the Quechua language of the ancient Inca empire, contains dimethyltryptamine (DMT), a chemical resembling the psilocybin compound in psychedelic mushrooms. DMT is the most powerful psychedelic compound known to man; it's produced naturally by the brain before death and might explain our reasons for believing in a glowing afterlife:

> The history of DMT dates back several hundred years when it started as a substance used during religious ceremonies and rituals. DMT is found in a number of South American-brewed concoctions like Ayahuasca. DMT can be produced synthetically, and its original synthesis was created by a British chemist in 1931 named Richard Manske. Only in recent years has it become a drug used for recreation and possibly associated with addiction...It is the strongest of all psychedelic drugs and is sometimes referred to as an "entheogen" a word that means "god-generated-within." The drug's chemical root structure is similar to that of the anti-migraine drug sumatriptan. It acts as a non-selective agonist at most or all of the serotonin receptors. DMT is not active when taken orally unless it is combined with another substance that inhibits its metabolism. The drug gained popularity in the 1960's and was placed under federal control under Schedule I when the Controlled Substances Act was passed in 1971...When combined in Ayahuasca, the presence of harmala alkaloids inhibits the enzyme monoamine oxidase, which normally metabolizes the tryptamine hallucinogen. Then the drug remains intact so that it absorbs in sufficient amounts to affect brain function and it results in psychoactive effects.[8]

The DMT that's absorbed into the ayahuasca brew is no joke, and unlike acid, which can be enjoyable, the purpose of an ayahuasca trip isn't to enjoy yourself—it's to journey inward for 24 hours, after puking and shitting your brains out. Leanna Standish, the neuroscientist who had a mind-bending ayahuasca experience in Brazil almost twenty years ago, has been trying to get scientific permission to study the therapeutic potentials of the trippy ancient vine. Finally, the FDA approved her protocol for the first trial in America using ayahuasca as a treatment for depression. Currently she's overseeing a facility in Hawaii that's growing the necessary plants needed for the ayahuasca tea when she plans to start her study in the summer of 2018. Standish, a professor at the Bastyr University Research Institute in Seattle, is joined by neuroscientist Jessica Nielson from the University of California-San Francisco, and Jordi Riba, a researcher at the Sant Pau Institute of Biomedical Research in Barcelona, as the leading psychedelic scientists challenging governments around the world to begin approving research into the therapeutic potentials of ayahuasca. Jordi is hoping to receive approval from the Spanish government for his study into ayahuasca as a PTSD treatment; if successful it will be the first ayahuasca therapeutic trial in Europe.

People from around the world travel to South America every year to drink ayahuasca for mental health issues including alcoholism, depression, anxiety, PTSD and drug addiction. Shamans also travel illegally with the holy ayahuasca and hold ceremonies in major cities across America, Australia, Canada, and Europe. Once a year a shaman from Venezuela comes to Homestead, outside of Miami, and conducts an elaborate ayahuasca ceremony, complete with a bonfire and romantic shits in the Everglades in the company of alligators. The ayahuasca brew is made from the bark of a vine called Banisteriopsis caapi which grows in the Amazon and the leaves of a shrub called Psychotria viridis, also native to the region. The psychedelic brew puts people in deep states of introspection that last for hours. Once they emerge back from the ethereal spirit world, they often report encounters with extradimensional lizard beings or encounters with spirit animals like jaguars. Overall most ayahuasca trips seem to have a long-lasting positive impact on those brave enough to take the ride. Unfortunately, there's only limited empirical data that suggest ayahuasca can be a helpful therapeutic drug, but thanks to a new breed of scientists, many of whom changed their minds about the drug after their own astounding ayahuasca experiences, are looking to change that.

Draulio Barros de Araujo, a professor of neuroimaging at the Brain Institute in Brazil, discovered that participants who tested ayahuasca for depression reported a 64% drop in symptoms one week later, after a single dose of the drug. But how did the shamans of the Amazon thousands of years ago know how to mix these two plants together to create the most complex psychedelic pharmacology in the world, while here we are, just now discovering it, and limiting it at the same time:

> The cultural and religious history of ayahuasca presents unique research questions. From a biomedical perspective, ayahuasca is just a drug—as long as a researcher has access to it, they can study it. But traditionally, ayahuasca is seen in South America as a sentient plant which heals when administered in a ceremony by a shaman or religious leader who is playing sacred songs and performing a number of other rituals. The ayahuasca researchers, many of whom have participated in ceremonies, respect these beliefs— and some think there is truth to them—but they're also bound by the rules of scientific investigation. If there are too many variables in their clinical trials, they'll be unable to produce consistent results or determine what aspect of the treatment was effective.[9]

Once again, the iron-fisted rule of the government hampers the ability of scientists and researchers willing to explore these new fields of psychedelic research by keeping psychedelics in the "drugs" category under the dreaded Schedule I act put into place almost fifty years ago. An act, by the way, that nobody voted on; it was passed in the dead of night and not in your favor. "You wanna get rid of drug crime in this country? Fine, let's just get rid of all the drug laws." Words of reason from Ron Paul, former congressmen, patriot and presidential candidate who was exposing the CIA's involvement in the drug war way back in the 1980s. But psychedelic drugs like LSD were never big moneymakers in the illegal drug game, like cocaine or even marijuana were, and so were left by the wayside after being declared illegal in the 1970s.

Even today, there's hardly a popping LSD market, so it's not like if psychedelics were suddenly made legal the crime cartels would lose any profit. Legalization would free up the medical world to explore all the possible therapeutic benefits psychedelics might achieve.

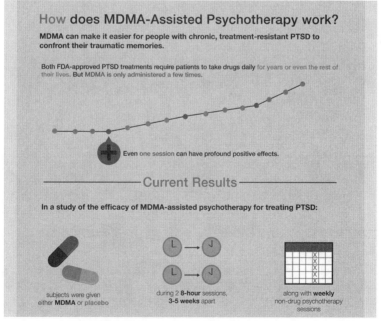

PTSD & MDMA (*American Infographic*)

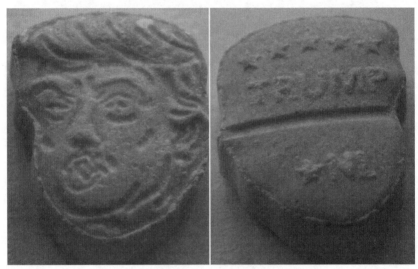

Trump inspired ecstasy tablets (*Reddit*)

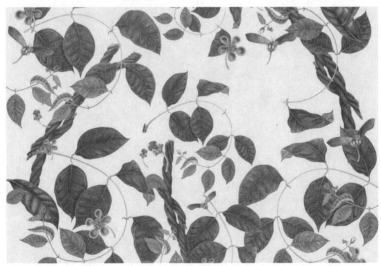

The Flowers and Vines of the Ayahuasca (*Donna Torres*)

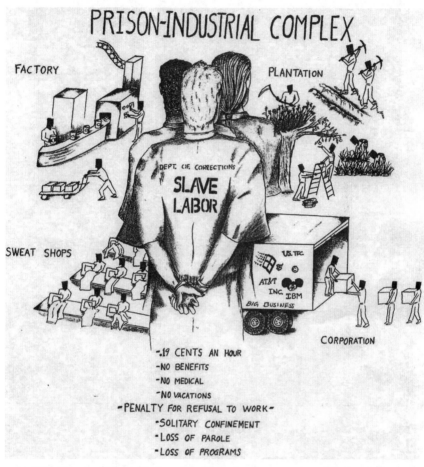

What is the Prison Industrial Complex? (*Empty Cages Collective*)

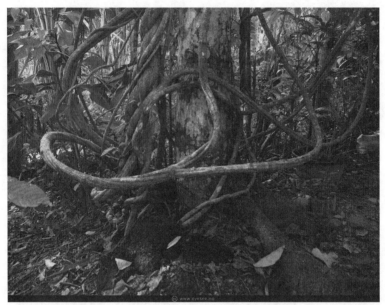

Ayahuasca growing in the wild (*Pinterest*)

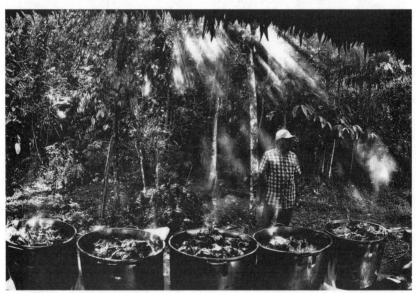

Pots containing the ingredients to make Ayahuasca (*abc.net.au*)

Chapter Twelve

The Healing Powers of Psychedelics

*Our society values alert problem solving
consciousness. And it devalues all other states of
consciousness. Any kind of consciousness that is not
related to the production or consumption of material
goods is stigmatized in our society today. Of course,
we accept drunkenness. We allow people some brief
respite from the material grind. A society that subscribes
to that model is a society that is going to condemn the
states of consciousness that have nothing to do with
the alert problem solving mentality. And if you go back
to the 1960's when there was a tremendous upsurge of
exploration of psychedelics, I would say that the huge
backlash that followed that had to do with a fear on the
part of the powers that be, that if enough people went into
those realms and those experiences the very fabric of the
society that we have today would be picked apart and
most importantly, those in power at the top would not be
in power at the top anymore.*
—Graham Hancock

A psychedelic utopia has been opposed and persecuted by authorities for centuries, both in Europe and in America. But we now know more than ever about what psychedelics do and how to utilize them in ways never imagined. "We didn't have as much data then as we do now," says Dr. Dan Engle, a board-certified psychiatrist, and avid psychedelic enthusiast. "And we didn't have as many of the safeguards as we have now. The psychedelic renaissance as a cornerstone in the redemption of modern psychiatric care...brain-network connections light up on psilocybin compared to the normal brain. More cross-regional firing. That's what the brain actually looks like on the 'drugs' that we've been using for hundreds if not thousands of years."[1]

Dr. Engle is talking about the scans that show where psilocybin interacts with certain regions of the brain as compared to images of the same areas without psychedelic highlights. These came from high-level psilocybin studies with extremely positive outcomes that remain largely ignored by the general medical communities and mainstream media. But those fortunate and rich enough don't need to wait around for clinical trials or hobo shamans, they can book an ayahuasca trip to Peru with Entrepreneurs Awakening, a California travel agency that arranges Peruvian tours of inner awakenings. Eric Weinstein, managing director at Thiel Capital in San Francisco, speaks from experience about these ayahuasca-themed tours and the power of the vine:

> These things are so powerful, that they can get into layers of patterned behavior to show folks things that they could change and could do differently. And the brain has probably been playing with these ideas in the subconscious. This entire family of agents is extraordinary, as they appear to be very profound, unexpectedly constructive and surprisingly safe. Most people who take these agents seem to discover cognitive modes that they never knew even existed.[2]

Weinstein wants to put together a series of public-service commercials in favor of legalizing psychedelics and has the support of other influential Silicon Valley luminaries and scientists like himself. However, a lot of super rich and privileged people that go full psychedelics usually end up getting all self-righteous and leave their multimillion-dollar companies to go do yoga and finance art and music projects that slowly drain all their resources, leaving them with a blown mind and lots to ponder. Super frat bro Chris Hunter, the 38-year-old inventor of the poisonous caffeinated maltliquor beverage *Four Loko*, went into his ayahuasca trip asking himself, "Why are you such a dick?" Hours later the response made him a new man. "What if you approached masculinity in a different way—instead of being dominant and overseeing the women in your life, you came from the other side, underneath, fully supporting and lifting women up?"[3] Words of advice from the man who created one of the world's most vilified products?

Research has shown that psychedelic treatments have led to people being better partners to their spouses, better parents to their children, and overall better human beings in general. Psychedelic therapy has gone underground, and the doctors brave enough to conduct their private trials have so far been left alone by the DEA, mostly because of the extreme wealth of the clientele. To dabble in the psychedelic world these days is far more expensive than it was in the hippie-drenched 60s. The *man*, it seems has other priorities than messing with doctors trying to heal the emotional wounds of a few rich people. Psychedelics are popular enough with the rich and famous, and even highly respected scientists, but it's when the average Joe has access to them that draws the line in establishment thinking for possible legalization. For the time being, the success stories show the importance of advocating to legalize psychedelics, so that we can study and use these plants and other medicines to save people's lives. The longer these drugs are kept illegal, the more chance the establishment has at breaking up families and sending more people to the prison slave factories. How many of our artistic heroes like the musician Prince could we have saved from opioid addiction with the help of psychedelic therapy?

Psychedelic drugs cause the brain to enter higher states of consciousness, a phenomenon long ridiculed but now admitted to exist by scientists. For the first time, science has shown the diversity of brain activity increasing because of taking psychedelic drugs. Scientists are hopeful the findings will lead to new treatments for depression and schizophrenia. Anil Seth, author of the study's report and co-director of the Sackler Centre for Consciousness Science at the University of Sussex in southern England, says:

[A higher state of consciousness] has a very specific meaning in terms of this study, and that meaning can get a little conflated with the hippy idea of a higher state of consciousness and psychedelic drugs. What we mean in this study is the measure of the mathematical diversity of brain activity, which, very roughly, is how unpredictable the activity of the brain is. We use this [because] this measure has previously been applied to try to track changes when people fall asleep or go under general anesthesia, which would generally be thought of as a lower state of consciousness. Boundaries between self and world disintegrate and things like that, we predicted that instead of a reduction in the level of diversity [as seen when you go to sleep], we'd see an increase. And that's what we found… it's higher on this specific scale of diversity, or unpredictability of the brain activity. This is the first example that I'm aware of where it goes in the other direction, where you see an increase in this measure.[4]

In 2014, Robin Carhart-Harris became the first person in the United Kingdom to administer LSD to humans for research purposes in over 40 years. In his study, published in 2016, scientists gave participants doses of LSD, ketamine and psilocybin and then looked at the participants' brain activity. The study showed what happens to people's brains on psychedelic drugs, providing a stunning series of technicolor images highlighting the event. The study not only showed how psychedelics alter brain changes, but also shows when the brain enters a higher state of consciousness. The scientists measured the magnetic fields produced by the brain in different states and found increased brain signal diversity when people were on psychedelic drugs, as opposed to when they were in a sober waking state. Carhart-Harris said, "People often say they experience insight under these [psychedelic] drugs—and when this occurs in a therapeutic context, it can predict positive outcomes. The present findings may help us understand how this can happen."[5] Your brain on psychedelic drugs is provenly different and shown to resonate higher on this specific one dimensional scale with a distinctive change in consciousness. These studies are striving to understand what's happening in the brain and what therapeutic effects can be obtained under psychedelic intoxication. From the study:

> In a new era of psychedelic research that's been restarted after many years alone in the wilderness, science is once again looking at the therapeutic uses of psychedelic

medicine. As our understanding of consciousness expands so does our desire to explore other avenues of non-traditional means to bring about change. When veterans are pilled to oblivion and don't have access to safer medications like marijuana and psychedelics they are far more at risk of committing suicide. Even though scientists don't exactly understand how or why psychedelic drugs provide significant benefits to people with depression, the evidence shows that they do. "Besides the fact that it actually changes [a depressed person's] experience of the world—it might kick them out of the ruminative tendencies and other things—we don't know why this is happening, there are clues. For instance, LSD works on the same chemical system in the brain that antidepressants work—the serotonin system. We know there's a pharmacological link, we know there's a change in experience and we know there's a clinical impact. But the middle bit if you like, what are these drugs doing to the global activity of the brain, that's the gap we're trying to fill with this study,"[6] says Anil Seth, one of the study's founders. Seth and his colleagues are the new breed of psychedelic pioneers looking to change the way people see the drug, hoping to fund research that better understands what happens to the brain when people are experiencing things like hallucinations. "If we can understand the brain basis of hallucinations then we'll understand a lot more about hallucinations—and not just about psychedelia but also in schizophrenia and other conditions," Seth says. "We'll also understand a lot more about how our visual experiences in the normal world happen. We're hallucinating all the time, it's just our hallucinations are usually controlled by the sensory data that we get."[7]

By observing the commonality in behaviors such as depression, anxiety, addiction, and OCD while under psychedelics, we can open up a window for therapeutic intervention which can recognize and replace the damaged behavioral patterns with more positive ones. Studies worldwide, both underground and clinical, all support the idea that psychedelics can have an extraordinarily positive effect on the future of therapy. After a single psychotherapy session with psilocybin, researchers at Johns Hopkins and NYU reported an 80% success rate in reducing anxiety and depression in terminal cancer patients. With each study, the extraordinary benefits of psychedelics become clearer and clearer. It's amazing to consider that merely a wee bit of psychedelia can have such long-lasting effects when most medicines are meant to be taken regularly and repeatedly, in order to maintain their effect. Most adults over the age of 40 take around 8 pills of various medicines on a daily basis. Imagine replacing those with a little bit of marijuana and magic mushrooms; guaranteed you'd be a lot healthier. Of course, the billions earned from the average pill-popping Joe is enough to keep the medical industrial complex in business for generations to come:

> If restrictions were lifted and more funding was available, we could undertake a much wider spectrum of research and consider their potential efficacy in many unexplored areas of healthcare, such as the ever increasing problem of dementia and Alzheimer's. We could also conduct the full clinical trials necessary to demonstrate beyond doubt that these drugs have therapeutic value, paving the way for them to be developed into life-changing medicines. As well as changing scheduling rules, we need to change the public perception of psychedelic drugs, which are often dominated by fear... a whole generation has been told that they're toxic and dangerous, and only ever harmful to mental health. It is true that they can be misused and cause harm, but this problem can't be solved by prohibition, and it certainly can't be solved by scheduling laws that prevent even basic research into their potential harms and benefits alike being carried out. There are many classes of drug which we accept can be prescribed and used responsibly by those in need of them, even though they also have the potential to be misused. For example, amphetamines are both prescribed as a treatment for ADHD and taken recreationally as a

stimulant. The opiate family includes both morphine, a useful painkiller, and heroin. There is nothing stopping us from taking the same attitude towards psychedelics: that with clinical oversight, their therapeutic benefits could vastly outweigh their risks.[8]

But alas, Big Pharma continues waging its war on psychedelics which is a war on all of us. Painfully unaware, too, are they of the great achievements already brought to the world thanks to the mind-expanding wonders of psychedelics.

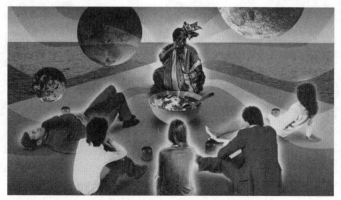

Ayahuasca treatments for the rich *(Be Well Buzz)*

191

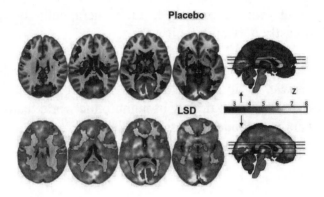

Scans showing marked difference in active areas between placebo and LSD (*New Scientist*)

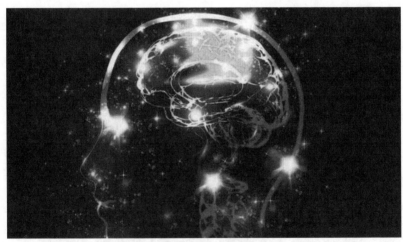

Your brain on LSD *(Pinterest)*

Chapter Thirteen

Great Achievements While Tripping

Deep in the human unconscious is a pervasive need for a logical universe that makes sense. But the real universe is always one step beyond logic... Without change something sleeps inside us, and seldom awakens. The sleeper must awaken.
—Frank Herbert, *Dune*

Frank Herbert wrote his classic sci-fi novel *Dune* while tripping on magic mushrooms. In fact the novel is basically an homage to the funky psychedelic, with the book's fictional spice, *mélange* (considered the most important commodity in the universe), acting in place of the sacred shroom. This naturally growing spice, which gives users heightened awareness, psychic powers and the ability to see into the future, can only be found on the planet Arrakis. The spice is also a power source for spaceships that are steered via navigational trances, but too much of the potent drug leads to addiction, turning users into luminous blue-eyed zombies that wither away from fatal withdrawals. At the time of *Dune*'s publication in 1965, many thought Herbert's "spice" was a reference to LSD. And in a way it was, as Herbert was writing about all psychedelics, in particular his own fondness for magic mushrooms. You see, Herbert was doing his own blue-ringed magic mushroom hunting in the Tacoma area long before most people even realized the legendary author was from there. Paul Stamets got to hang out with Herbert during research for his book *Mycelium Running: How Mushrooms Can Help Save the World*:

Frank Herbert, the well-known author of the Dune books, told me his technique for using spores. When I met

193

him in the early 1980s, Frank enjoyed collecting mushrooms on his property near Port Townsend, Washington. An avid mushroom collector, he felt that throwing his less-than-perfect wild chanterelles into the garbage or compost didn't make sense. Instead, he would put a few weathered chanterelles in a 5-gallon bucket of water, add some salt, and then, after 1 or 2 hours, pour this spore-mass slurry on the ground at the base of newly planted firs. When he told me chanterelles were growing from trees not even 10 years old, I couldn't believe it. No one had previously reported chanterelles arising near such young trees, nor had anyone reported them growing as a result of using this method. Of course, it did work for Frank, who was simply following nature's lead. Frank's discovery has now been confirmed in the mushroom industry. It is now known that it's possible to grow many mushrooms using spore slurries from elder mushrooms. Many variables come into play, but in a sense this method is just a variation of what happens when it rains. Water dilutes spores from mushrooms and carries them to new environments. Our responsibility is to make that path easier. Such is the way of nature. Frank went on to tell me that much of the premise of *Dune*—the magic spice (spores) that allowed the bending of space (tripping), the giant worms (maggots digesting mushrooms), the eyes of the Freman (the cerulean blue of Psilocybe mushrooms), the mysticism of the female spiritual warriors, the Bene Gesserits (influenced by tales of Maria Sabina and the sacred mushroom cults of Mexico)—came from his perception of the fungal life cycle, and his imagination was stimulated through his experiences with the use of magic mushrooms.[1]

Francis Crick, the Nobel Prize winning biologist, biophysicist, and neuroscientist, discovered DNA while tripping on LSD in 1953. This landmark event in the human history of genetics, made Francis Crick a science-nerd rock star, even though his peers never knew LSD was involved in his discovery until decades later. When Crick came bursting through the door to his home in Cambridge, babbling to his wife about two spirals twisting in opposite directions from one another and other jibberish, his wife, an artist, drew what her husband described. They then went out to celebrate at the pub even though Crick's wife, Odile, had no idea what they were celebrating. Far away was the idea that her drawing of twisty spirals would become one of the most reproduced illustrations in the history of science—a first draft of the double helix structure of DNA that scientists still refer to today. But Crick, when not discovering the key to life and winning prestigious prizes for doing so, spent the 50s and 60s throwing all night parties famous for LSD, vintage forms of bondage and nudity. The parties stopped when LSD became illegal, and although Crick never admitted publicly that he was on LSD when he figured out the double helix structure, his closest colleagues always knew, verifying the legend as true in 2006:

> The double helix is essentially the Sgt. Peppers of scientific models, a ladder that's been melted and twirled by a pasta fork, or the two snakes from the caduceus if one of them was fucking the other with 100 dicks (depending on whether the artist ate the good or bad acid). Now obviously scientists don't arrive at models by doodling on their trapper keeper and picking out the shape that looks the coolest. To do what Crick did required an insane amount of analytical, theoretical, and spatial thinking. It's not like Crick dropped out of high school and then used acid to turn himself into a supergenius. Crick was a fan of Aldous Huxley's *The Doors of Perception*, a study of the human mind which was undertaken like all good studies, while driving around LA on mescaline. Huxley wrote that the sober mind has a series of filters on it that basically prevent abstract thought (evolution put them there for the sake of survival, since having daydreams about the nature of the universe while driving can cause you to plow into a semi). But Huxley and Crick thought drugs like mescaline and LSD could temporarily remove those filters. So rather than melting his mind into a lava lamp of trippy shapes, Crick probably used LSD to get unfiltered access to a part

of his brain most normal people rarely use.[2]

Crick was also a fan of the ancient alien theory and believed that life was started on Earth by a race of prehistoric aliens, a controversial theory that isn't new to users of psychedelics, who are typically more open-minded than most people and willing to ponder the deepest truths of the universe despite how frightening they might seem. The fact that the discoverer of DNA was a fan of LSD and ancient aliens should let people know that psychedelics aren't dangerous despite being polarizing. Kary Mullis, another DNA pioneer, thought up the PCR (polymerase chain reaction, used for copying DNA) while also tripping on acid. But it's not just writers and scientists that have made breakthroughs in their works while under the influence of psychedelics. In the 1970s the Pittsburgh Pirates ballslinger Dock Ellis somehow tripped his way to a no-hitter.

Baseball is America's pastime and has been around seemingly forever, with more than half a million games played in MLB history. Surprisingly, there have been fewer than 250 of those in which the starting pitcher recorded every out without giving up a hit. Most pitchers, even the great ones, go their entire careers without throwing one. Hell, it even took the Mets more than fifty years and 8,000 games before the franchise logged their first no-hitter. So, how the hell did Dock Ellis became one of the few to ever do it—while tripping on acid?! On the day of the no-hitter, Dock Ellis woke up around noon unsure of what day it was, and ditched his bowl of *Wheaties* for three tabs of acid. By the time he got around to reading the sports section he found out that he was scheduled to pitch in San Diego in six hours, which was a surprise to him since he thought it was his day off. Ellis had thought the worst of his trip would be sitting around bored in the dugout waiting for the game to finish. No way was he prepared to pitch, especially after eating three hits of acid. But Ellis was used to pitching high, at least on speed and cocaine, which wasn't really a big deal to the league back in the 70s. Dock was known as the "king of speed" to his Pirate teammates, who often took bets on whether anyone could outdo him in the speed and cocaine baseball Olympics. But despite being a pro when it came to pitching under the influence of uppers and alcohol, Ellis had never even thought about having to play ball while at floating on psychedelics. Unfazed, Ellis hopped a flight to San Diego, and intensely chopped down a lineup that wasn't on acid to the point where no one got a single hit. Ellis remembers very little about the game, other than being in the zone and that sometimes the ball felt so huge in his hands while other times felt so tiny. Also that at one point he dove out of the way of a laser-like line drive that had barely dribbled back to the pitcher's mound. Somehow Ellis managed to pull himself together by muscle memory and intense concentration, tripping his way into the zone to pitch a better game than some of the greats like Pedro Martinez, Greg Maddux and Grover Cleveland Alexander ever did:

> A large part of throwing a no-hitter is getting over the fact that you're throwing one. As the game goes on and the lonely bastard in the middle of the diamond gets closer to immortality, the tension in the park and in the pitcher builds. Trying to throw a no-hitter is such a mind fuck that it's considered the height of dickery for a teammate to acknowledge the no-hitter until the final out is recorded. But baseball history was the last thing on Ellis' mind, keeping his shit together while a bunch of giant lizards fucked in the on-deck circle being the first. Ellis had the career trajectory of Darryl Strawberry, never reaching his potential because of drug addiction. Instead of being a household name, Dock Ellis is just that guy who threw a no-hitter on acid.[3]

Some of the most creative minds of our time partly credit their breakthroughs to psychedelics unlocking the mind-melting pathways to success. Whether it's in the fields of science, the arts or industry, the psychedelic-fueled voyage through inner space has proven useful to some people at the pinnacle of their fields. We've already spoken about how LSD led the Beatles to forever alter music history; meanwhile Cary Grant, the classic Hollywood leading man, repeatedly used LSD throughout his acting career. Grant credits LSD with bringing him happiness and helping him overcome the mental traumas suffered from an impoverished chaotic upbringing. In *Look* magazine's 1959 article "The Curious Story Behind the New Cary Grant," Grant talked positively about his acid therapy, saying, "I wanted to rid myself of all my hypocrisies. I wanted to work through the events of my childhood, my relationship with my parents and my former wives. I did not want to spend years in analysis."[4] He wanted to find happiness, and according to Grant himself, the LSD treatment therapies helped him achieve it.

Steve Jobs, Apple co-founder, legendary asshole, and one of the great entrepreneurial minds of contemporary times, loved munching on acid for a period of four transformative years. Jobs was deeply moved by his psychedelic experiences saying:

Throughout that period of time [1972-1974] I used the LSD approximately ten to fifteen times. I would ingest the LSD on a sugar cube or in a hard form of gelatin. I would usually take the LSD when I was by myself. I have no words to explain the effect the LSD had on me, although, I can say it was a positive life-changing experience for me and I am glad I went through that experience. Taking LSD was a profound experience, one of the most important things in my life. LSD shows you that there's another side to the coin, and you can't remember it when it wears off, but you know it. It reinforced my sense of what was important—creating great things instead of making money, putting things back into the stream of history and of human consciousness as much as I could.[5]

A host of philosophers also had positive experiences with psychedelics. Gerald Heard, a British author who wrote over thirty books on science, history, and human consciousness, tried LSD in the early 1950s. His societal influence caused the drug to be examined by fellow intellectual adventurers who also experienced moments of intense insight caused by the drug. Because of Heard, other psychedelic luminaries like Aldous Huxley and Timothy Leary volunteered to try LSD. His work had a tremendous influence on the consciousness development movement that arose in the West in the 1960s. Heard felt that, if used properly,

LSD had a strong potential to "enlarge man's mind" by allowing the individual to see beyond their own ego. In 1956, Alcoholics Anonymous founder Bill Wilson first took LSD under Heard's guidance and, according to Wilson, the session provided a spiritual experience that led him to overcome his alcohol addiction. Rare television footage of Heard discussing the drug with Dr. Sidney Cohen in Los Angeles in 1956 can be seen on Youtube. The section of Heard's discussion on LSD can be read below:

Dr Cohen: Now Gerald I know you have great personal experience with lysergic acid. What do you think of it?

Gerald Heard: To do this in two minutes, eternity in an hour. It's almost impossible of course as all the patients say to describe it. You can only say, "it isn't it isn't it isn't," trying to tell people what it is. Well of course, I don't know any of our friends said that have taken it but haven't said this one thing in common: "Well, I never knew anything like that in the whole of my life." And one or two people have said to me, I've said it to myself: "That's what death is going to be like. And oh what fun it will be."

Dr. Cohen: How do you mean that?

Gerald Heard: Well I mean that there are the colors and the beauties, the designs, the beautiful wavy things appear. People themselves—dull people that I thought dull appear fascinating interesting mysterious wonderful. But that's only the beginning. Man was saying it this afternoon who was taking it. Suddenly you notice that there aren't these separations. That we're not on a separate island shouting across to somebody else and trying to hear what they're saying and misunderstanding them. You know. You use the word yourself: empathy. These things flowing underneath. We're parts of a single continent. It meets underneath the water. And with that goes such delight. The sober certainty of waking bliss.[6]

Believing that it offered a positive way to help individuals understand the role their lives played in the universe, Alan Watts, another influential British philosopher best known for popularizing eastern philosophies to Western audiences, also experimented with LSD. "One of my earliest experiences with LSD was also one of my most powerful and transformative. At the peak, I was unable to tell whether I had my eyes open or closed, and I remember thinking to myself, 'If there is no difference between the inside and the outside, where am I?'"[7]

In 1968, Watts wrote a lengthy essay for the *California Law Review* describing his views on psychedelics, ridiculous drug laws, shamans and religion, and the various times he tripped:

> I myself have experimented with five of the principal psychedelics: LSD-25, mescaline, psilocybin, dimethyl-tryptamine (DMT), and cannabis. I have done so, as William James tried nitrous oxide, to see if they could help me in identifying what might be called the "essential" or "active" ingredients of the mystical experience...It struck me, therefore, that if any of the psychedelic chemicals would in fact predispose my consciousness to the mystical experience, I could use them as instruments for studying and describing that experience as one uses a microscope for bacteriology, even though the microscope is an "artificial" and "unnatural" contrivance which might be said to "distort" the vision of the naked eye. However, when I was first invited to test the mystical qualities of LSD-25 by Dr. Keith Ditman of the Neuropsychiatric Clinic at UCLA Medical School, I was unwilling to believe that any mere chemical could induce a genuine mystical experience. At most, it might bring about a state of spiritual insight analogous to swimming with water wings. Indeed, my first experiment with LSD-25 was not mystical. It was an intensely interesting aesthetic and intellectual experience that challenged my powers of analysis and careful description to the utmost. Some months later, in 1959, I tried LSD-25 again with Drs. Sterling Bunnell and Michael Agron, who were then associated with the Langley-Porter Clinic, in San Francisco. In the course of two experiments I was amazed and somewhat embarrassed to find myself going through states of consciousness that corresponded

precisely with every description of major mystical experiences that I had ever read. Through subsequent experimentation with LSD-25 and the other chemicals named above (with the exception of DMT, which I find amusing but relatively uninteresting), I found I could move with ease into the state of "cosmic consciousness," and in due course became less and less dependent on the chemicals themselves for "tuning in" to this particular wave length of experience. Of the five psychedelics tried, I found that LSD-25 and cannabis suited my purposes best. Of these two, the latter—cannabis—which I had to use abroad in countries where it is not outlawed, proved to be the better.[8]

Alan Watts was unaware that his clinical stash of LSD had arrived via the CIA, as most people at the time, even the doctors running the trials, were also unaware. Modern philosophers like Chris Letheby believe that psychedelic drugs are a legitimate way to achieve spiritual and therapeutic transformations, and they are. But only when they are removed from the Schedule I illegal listing will we be able to truly enjoy the psychedelic utopia first dreamed about by philosophers, mystics and writers—way before the CIA let their little liquid conspiracy get out of hand. Imagine how different the world would be if psychedelics weren't made illegal in the 1970s. The outcome of life for many would have been a helluva lot different if the agency decided to disperse LSD in the ghettos of the 80s instead of crack cocaine.

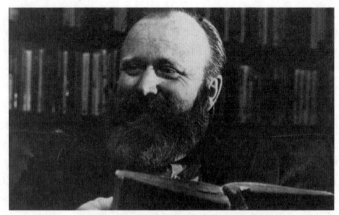

Frank Herbert (*Reality Sandwich*)

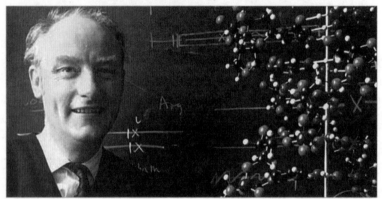

Francis Crick (*io9*)

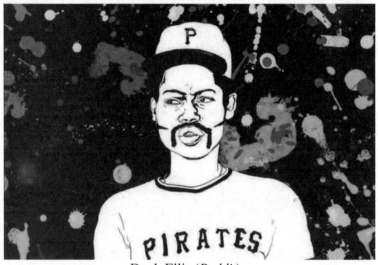

Dock Ellis (*Reddit*)

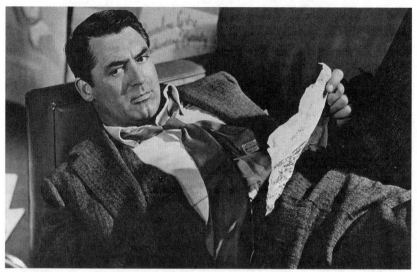

Cary Grant (*Pinterest*)

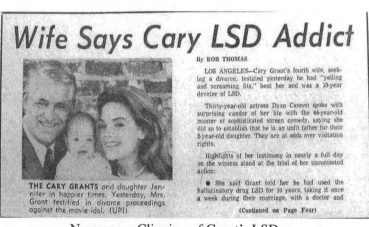

Wife Says Cary LSD Addict

By BOB THOMAS

LOS ANGELES—Cary Grant's fourth wife, seeking a divorce, testified yesterday he had "yelling and screaming fits," beat her and was a 10-year devotee of LSD.

Thirty-year-old actress Dyan Cannon spoke with surprising candor of her life with the 64-year-old master of sophisticated screen comedy, saying she did so to establish that he is an unfit father for their 2-year-old daughter. They are at odds over visitation rights.

Highlights of her testimony in nearly a full day on the witness stand at the trial of her uncontested action:

● She said Grant told her he had used the hallucinatory drug LSD for 10 years, taking it once a week during their marriage, with a doctor and

THE CARY GRANTS and daughter Jennifer in happier times. Yesterday, Mrs. Grant testified in divorce proceedings against the movie idol. (UPI)

(Continued on Page Four)

Newspaper Clipping of Grant's LSD use

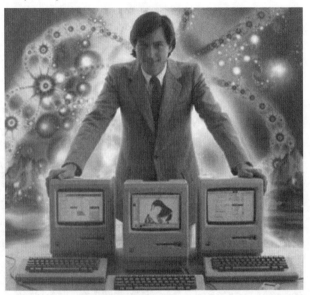

Steve Jobs (*Forbes*)

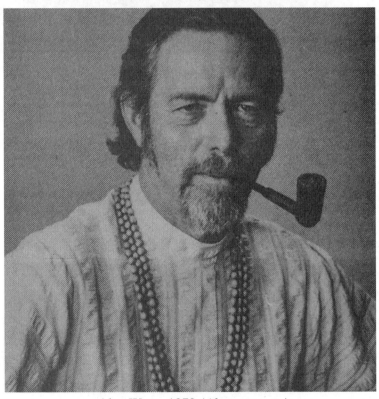

Alan Watts, 1970 (*Alanwatts.org*)

NOTES

Introduction
1. Albert Hofmann, *LSD: My Problem Child*, Oxford University Press, London, 1976
2. Michael Horowitz, "Interview with Albert Hofmann," *High Times*, 1976, https://erowid.org/culture/characters/hofmann_albert/hofmann_albert_interview1.shtml
3. "Senate Report hearings on testing and use of chemical and biological agents by the intelligence communities," http://www.turnerhome.org/jct/Church-1.html
4. Andrei Codrescu, "Whose Worlds are These?," Introduction to *Acid Dreams*, Grove Press, New York, 1985

The Pioneers of Psychedelia
1. "Aldous Huxley: L.A. Writer," *American Legends*, http://americanlegends.com/authors/aldous_huxley.html
2. Martin A. Lee and Bruce Shlain, *Acid Dreams: The Complete Social History of LSD: The CIA, the Sixties and Beyond*, Grove Press, New York, 1985, http://www.levity.com/aciddreams/samples/history.html
3. Ibid
4. Tyler Durden, "Prison States of America," *Zero Hedge*, December 30, 2014, http://www.zerohedge.com/news/2014-12-30/prison-state-america

Operations Bluebird and Artichoke
1. Martin A. Lee and Bruce Shlain, *Acid Dreams: The Complete Social History of LSD: The CIA, the Sixties and Beyond,* Grove Press, New York, 1985
2. "Project CHATTER," *Wikispooks*, https://wikispooks.com/wiki/Project_CHATTER
3. Martin A. Lee and Bruce Shlain, *Acid Dreams: The Complete Social History of LSD: The CIA, the Sixties and Beyond*, Grove Press, New York, 1985
4. "Project ARTICHOKE," *Wikispooks*, https://wikispooks.com/wiki/Project_ARTICHOKE
5. Martin A. Lee and Bruce Shlain, *Acid Dreams: The Complete Social History of LSD: The CIA, the Sixties and Beyond*, Grove Press, New York, 1985
6. Ibid
7. Ibid

8. Ibid
9. Ibid
10. Ibid
11. Ibid

Daytrippers: The CIA's Mad LSD Scientists
1. Jordan Todorov, "The Early, State-Sanctioned LSD Experiments in Communist Bulgaria," *Atlas Obscura*, May 25, 2016, http://www.atlasobscura.com/articles/the-early-state-sanctioned-lsd-experiments-in-communist-bulgaria
2. Ibid
3. Richard Stratton, "Government Mind Control Agent Talks MK-ULTRA, the CIA, and LSD," *Whowhatwhy.org*, April 29, 2016, https://whowhatwhy.org/2016/04/29/government-mind-control-agent-talks/
4. Martin A. Lee and Bruce Shlain, *Acid Dreams: The Complete Social History of LSD: The CIA, the Sixties and Beyond*, Grove Press, New York, 1985
5. Nick Allen, "How Uri Geller convinced the CIA he was a 'psychic warrior,'" *Telegraph*, January 18, 2017, http://www.telegraph.co.uk/news/2017/01/18/uri-geller-convinced-cia-psychic-warrior/
6. Ibid
7. Martin A. Lee and Bruce Shlain, *Acid Dreams: The Complete Social History of LSD: The CIA, the Sixties and Beyond*, Grove Press, New York, 1985
8. "The CIA's obsession with LSD in the water supply," *Boingboing.net*, https://boingboing.net/2010/08/20/the-cias-obsession-w.html
9. Ibid
10. "William Millarc," *Newspapers*, https://www.newspapers.com/newspage/67399818/
11. "Secret London: LSD experiments at the World Psychedelic Centre," *Great Wen*, November 30, 2011, https://greatwen.com/2011/11/30/secret-london-lsd-experiments-at-the-world-psychedelic-centre/
12. Martin A. Lee and Bruce Shlain, *Acid Dreams: The Complete Social History of LSD: The CIA, the Sixties and Beyond*, Grove Press, New York, 1985
13. Ibid
14. Ibid

15. Ibid
16. Ibid
17. Ibid
18. Ibid

Timothy Leary, Harvard and the LSD Beatniks
1. Timothy Leary, *High Priest*, New American Library, New York, 1968
2. Ibid
3. Martin A. Lee and Bruce Shlain, *Acid Dreams: The Complete Social History of LSD: The CIA, the Sixties and Beyond*, Grove Press, New York, 1985
4. Ibid
5. Ibid
6. Ibid
7. William S. Burroughs, *Nova Express*, Grove Press, New York, 1964
8. Martin A. Lee and Bruce Shlain, *Acid Dreams: The Complete Social History of LSD: The CIA, the Sixties and Beyond*, Grove Press, New York, 1985
9. Timothy Leary, *High Priest*, New American Library, New York, 1968
10. Martin A. Lee and Bruce Shlain, *Acid Dreams: The Complete Social History of LSD: The CIA, the Sixties and Beyond*, Grove Press, New York, 1985
11. Ibid
12. Ibid
13. Ibid
14. Ibid

Taste the Electric Kool Aid: Ken Kesey's Magic Bus Ride

1. Martin A. Lee and Bruce Shlain, *Acid Dreams: The Complete Social History of LSD: The CIA, the Sixties and Beyond*, Grove Press, New York, 1985
2. Ibid
3. Sterling Lord, "When Kerouac Met Kesey," *The American Scholar*, 2011, https://theamericanscholar.org/when-kerouac-met-kesey/#
4. Martin A. Lee and Bruce Shlain, *Acid Dreams: The Complete Social History of LSD: The CIA, the Sixties and Beyond*,

Grove Press, New York, 1985
5. Ibid
6. Ibid
7. Ibid
8. Ibid
9. Ibid

The MIC, CIA and the Wizards of Laurel Canyon

1. Dave McGowan, "Inside The LC: The Strange but Mostly True Story of Laurel Canyon and the Birth of the Hippie Generation Part 1," *The Center for an Informed America*, 2008, https://www.sott.net/article/155794-Inside-The-LC-The-Strange-but-Mostly-True-Story-of-Laurel-Canyon-and-the-Birth-of-the-Hippie-Generation-Part-1
2. "H.H. Wilcox," *Wikipedia*, https://en.wikipedia.org/wiki/Harvey_Henderson_Wilcox
3. "The Wizard of Hollywood," *Motor Age*, Volume 5, pp. 133
4. Jordan Maxwell, *Matrix of Power*, The Book Tree, San Diego, California, 2000
5. Diane Wedner, "Hiking into Hollywood's backyard," *Los Angeles Times*, June 1, 2008, http://articles.latimes.com/2008/jun/01/realestate/re-guide1
6. Dave McGowan, "Inside The LC: The Strange but Mostly True Story of Laurel Canyon and the Birth of the Hippie Generation Part 1," *The Center for an Informed America*, 2008
7. "Declassified Charlton Heston Government Film: Trust But Verify," *Youtube*, https://www.youtube.com/watch?v=utHfA4vJVYc
8. "Zappa on LSD," *LSD Wiki*, http://wiki.killuglyradio.com/wiki/LSD
9. Dave McGowan, "Inside The LC: The Strange but Mostly True Story of Laurel Canyon and the Birth of the Hippie Generation Part 1," *The Center for an Informed America*, 2008
10. Ibid
11. Ibid

The MI6, The Beatles and LSD

1. Legs McNeil and Gillian McCain, "The Oral History of the First Two Times the Beatles Took Acid," *Vice*, December

4, 2016, https://www.vice.com/en_us/article/ppawq9/the-oral-history-of-the-beatles-first-two-acids-trips-legs-mcneil-gillian-mccain

2. Ibid
3. Ibid
4. Ibid
5. Ibid
6. Ibid
7. Ibid
8. Ibid
9. Ibid
10. Mikal Gilmore, "Inside the Making of 'Sgt. Pepper,'" *Rolling Stone*, June 1, 2017, http://www.rollingstone.com/music/features/inside-the-making-of-the-beatles-sgt-pepper-w484129
11. "Playboy Interview with John Lennon and Yoko Ono," *Beatlesinterviews.org*, http://www.beatlesinterviews.org/dbjypb.int3.html
12. Rob Evans, "Drugged and duped," *Guardian*, March 14, 2002, https://www.theguardian.com/education/2002/mar/14/research.highereducation
13. Ibid
14. Ibid
15. Ibid

LSD Over Pont-Saint-Esprit and the Rise of Psychedelic Cinema

1. Henry Samuel, "French bread spiked with LSD in CIA experiment," *Telegraph*, March 11, 2010, http://www.telegraph.co.uk/news/worldnews/europe/france/7415082/French-bread-spiked-with-LSD-in-CIA-experiment.html
2. Ibid
3. Ibid
4. Jeff Stafford, "Easy Rider TCM," *TCM*, http://www.tcm.com/this-month/article/188869%7C0/Easy-Rider.html

Scopolamine: The CIA's Real Truth Serum

1. George Bimmerle, "'Truth' Drugs in Interrogation," *CIA.gov*, https://www.cia.gov/library/center-for-the-study-of-intelligence/kent-csi/vol5no2/html/v05i2a09p_0001.htm
2. Dan Goodin, "Body of murdered cyberwar expert found

in landfill," *The Register*, January 5, 2011, https://www.theregister.co.uk/2011/01/05/cyberwar_expert_homicide/

3. "Soviet Use of Assassination and Kidnapping," *CIA.gov*, https://www.cia.gov/library/center-for-the-study-of-intelligence/kent-csi/vol19no3/html/v19i3a01p_0001.htm

4. "Drugs used in mind control quotes," *Whale.to*, http://www.whale.to/b/drugs1.html

The Magic Mushrooms at the End of the Rainbow

1. Brigit Katz, "Scientists unlock magic mushrooms mysterious chemical compound," *Smithsonian Magazine*, August 15, 2017, http://www.smithsonianmag.com/smart-news/scientists-unlock-magic-mushrooms-mysterious-chemical-compound-180964552/

2. Ibid

3. Ibid

4. Ibid

5. Ibid

6. "Exodus 16:14," *Bible Hub*, http://biblehub.com/exodus/16-14.htm

7. John Allegro, *The Sacred Mushroom and the Cross*, Hodder & Stoughton Ltd, London, 1970

8. Ibid

9. Janet Burns, "Global Survey Says Magic Mushrooms Are The Safest Recreational Drug," *Forbes*, May 26, 2017, https://www.forbes.com/sites/janetwburns/2017/05/26/global-survey-says-magic-mushrooms-are-the-safest-recreational-drug/#17e734014dad

Big Pharma's War on Psychedelics

1. Melly Alazraki, "Health Insurer Profits Jumped 250% in Last Decade," *AOL*, Febuary 18, 2010, https://www.aol.com/2010/02/18/health-insurer-profits-jumped-250-in-last-decade/

2. Stephie Grob Plante, "The war on drugs is back. Will psychedelic drug research survive?," *The Verge*, June 28, 2017, https://www.theverge.com/2017/6/28/15880260/trump-jeff-sessions-fda-mdma-psychedelic-drug-safety-research

3. Ibid

4. Mac McClelland, "How some doctors are risking everything to unleash the healing power of MDMA, ayahuasca and other

hallucinogens," *Rolling Stone*, March 9, 2017, http://www.
rollingstone.com/culture/features/how-doctors-treat-mental-
illness-with-psychedelic-drugs-w470673
5. Ibid
6. Ibid
7. Ibid
8. "The Most Powerful Psychedelic Drug: What is DMT and
   What are the Effects?," *The Recovery Village*, https://www.
   therecoveryvillage.com/dmt-addiction/#gref
9. Shelby Hartman, "The ayahuasca ceremony is going under
   the scientific-method microscope," *Quartz*, April 20, 2017,
   https://qz.com/963683/the-ayahuasca-ceremony-is-going-
   under-the-scientific-method-microscope/

The Healing Powers of Psychedelics
1. Mac McClelland, "How some doctors are risking everything
   to unleash the healing power of MDMA, ayahuasca and other
   hallucinogens," *Rolling Stone*, March 9, 2017, http://www.
   rollingstone.com/culture/features/how-doctors-treat-mental-
   illness-with-psychedelic-drugs-w470673
2. Ibid
3. Ibid
4. Ibid
5. L. Carhart-Harris, etc., "Neural correlates of the LSD
   experience revealed by multimodal neuroimaging," *Pnas.org*,
   March 1, 2016, http://www.pnas.org/content/113/17/4853.
   long
6. Hannah Osborne, "Psychedelic Drugs: The Brain Enters a
   'Higher State of Consciousness' on LSD and Ketamine,"
   Newsweek, April 4, 2017, http://www.newsweek.
   com/psychedelic-drugs-lsd-ketamine-brain-higher-
   consciousness-586076
7. Ibid
8. Amanda Fielding, "The Future of Psychedelic Medicine,"
   Huffington Post UK, January 17, 2017, http://www.
   huffingtonpost.co.uk/amanda-feilding/the-future-of-
   psychedelic_b_14144246.htm

Great Achievements While Tripping
1. Jeremy D. Johnson, "Magic Mushrooms Inspired Frank
   Herbert's *Dune*," *Reality Sandwich*, July 25, 2014, http://

   realitysandwich.com/221354/magic-mushrooms-inspired-the-spice-behind-frank-herberts-dune/
2. Jack O'Brien, "The 5 Greatest Things Ever Accomplished While High," *Cracked*, August 4, 2008, http://www.cracked.com/article_16532_the-5-greatest-things-ever-accomplished-while-high.html
3. Ibid
4. Philip Smith, "7 People Who Say They Owe Their Huge Success to Psychedelics," *Alternet.org*, January 26, 2015, http://www.alternet.org/drugs/seven-high-achievers-credit-psychedelics-their-success
5. Ibid
6. "Philosopher Gerald Heard on LSD," *Youtube*, https://www.youtube.com/watch?v=1pI5XZxpQaI
7. Alan Watts, "Psychedelics and Religious Experience," *Psychedelic-library.org*, http://www.psychedelic-library.org/watts.htm
8. Ibid

Bibliography

Aaronson, Bernard and Osmond, Humphrey, eds. *Psychedelics: The Uses and Implications of Hallucinogenic Drugs*. New York: Doubleday, 1970.

Abramson, Harold, ed. *The Use of LSD in Psychotherapy*. New York: The Josiah Macy, Jr. Foundation, 1960.

Abramson, Harold, ed. *The Use of LSD in Psychotherapy and Alcoholism*. Indianapolis: Bobbs-Merrill, 1967.

Agee, Philip. *Inside the Company: CIA Diary*. New York: Stonehill, 1975.

Aldiss, Brian. *Barefoot in the Head*. New York: Avon, 1981.

Allegro, John. *The Sacred Mushroom and the Cross*. London: Hodner and Stoughton, 1970.

Alpert, Richard. *Be Here Now*. San Cristobal, New Mexico: Lama Foundation, 1971.

Alpert, Richard, Cohen, Sidney, and Schiller, Lawrence. *LSD*. New York: New American Library, 1966.

Anderson, Chester. *The Butterfly Kid*. New York: Pocket Books, 1980.

Andrews, George and Vinkenoog, Simon., eds. *The Book of Grass*. New York: Grove Press, 1967.

Anson, Robert Sam. *Gone Crazy and Back Again*. New York: Doubleday, 1981.

Anthony, Gene. *The Summer of Love*. Millbrae, California: Celestial Arts, 1980.

Armstrong, David. *A Trumpet to Arms: Alternative Media in America*. Los Angeles: J.P. Tarcher, 1981.

Artaud, Antonin. *The Peyote Dance*. New York: Farrar, Straus and Giroux, 1976.

Ashbery, John. *Three Poems*. New York: Viking, 1975.

Baudelaire, Charles. *Artificial Paradise*. New York: Herder and Herder, 1971.

Beck, Julian. The Life of the Theatre. San Francisco: City Lights, 1972.

Bedford, Sybille. *Aldous Huxley, A Biography*. New York: Alfred A. Knopf, 1975.

Blum, Ralph. *The Simultaneous Man*. New York: Bantam, 1971.

Blum, Richard, and associates. *Utopiates: The Use and Users of LSD-2J*. New York: Atherton Press, 1965.

Booth, Stanley. *Dance with the Devil*. New York: Random House, 1984.

Bowart, Walter H. *Operation Mind Control*. New York: Dell, 1978.

Braden, William. *The Age of Aquarius*. New York: Pocket Books, 1971.

Braden, William. *The Private Sea: LSD and the Search for God*. New York: Bantam, 1968.

Breines, Wini. *Community & Organization in the New Left, 1962-1968: The Great Refusal*. South Hadley, Massachusetts: J.F. Bergin Publishers, 1982.

Breton, André. *What is Surrealism? Selected Writings. Franklin Rosemont*, ed. New York: Monad Press, 1978.

Brown, Anthony Cave. *Wild Bill Donovan: The Last Hero*. New York: Times Books, 1982.

Brown, Peter, and Gaines, Steven. *The Love You Make: An Insider's Story of the Beatles*. New York: Signet, 1983.

Browning, Frank, and the editors of *Ramparts. Smack!* New York: Harper &. Row, 1972.

Bryan, John. *What Ever Happened to Timothy Leary?* San Francisco: Renaissance Press, 1980.

Burroughs, William S. *The fob*. New York: Grove Press, 1974.

Burroughs, William S. *Naked Lunch*. New York: Grove Press, 1966.

Burroughs, William S. *Nova Express*. New York: Grove Press, 1965.

Burroughs, William S., and Ginsberg, Allen. *The Yage Letters*. San Francisco: City Lights, 1963.

Bylinsky, Gene. *Mood Control*. New York: Charles Scribner's Sons, 1978.

Caldwell, W V. *LSD Psychotherapy*. New York: Grove Press, 1969.

Carey, James T. *The College Drug Scene*. Englewood Cliffs, New Jersey: Prentice- Hall, 1968.

Case, John, and Taylor, Rosemary C.R., eds. Co-ops, *Communes & Collectives: Experiments in Social Change in the 1960s and 1970s*. New York: Pantheon, 1979.

Cashman, John. The LSD Story. Greenwich, Connecticut: Fawcett Publishers, 1966.

Castenada, Carlos. *The Teachings of Don Juan—A Yaqui Way of Knowledge*. Berkeley: University of California Press, 1968.

Charbonneau, Louis. *Psychedelic-40*. New York: Bantam, 1965.

Charters, Ann, ed. *The Beats: Literary Bohemians in Postwar America* (Vols. I and II). Detroit: Gale Research Company, 1973.

Chavkin, Samuel. *The Mind Stealers*. Boston: Houghton Mifflin, 1978.

Cholden, Louis, ed. *Lysergic Acid Diethylamide and Mescaline in Experimental Psychiatry*. New York: Grune & Stratton, 1956.

Clark, Walter Houston. *Chemical Ecstasy.* New York: Sheed and Ward, 1969.

Cleaver, Eldridge. *Soul on Ice*. New York: Dell, 1968.

Cohen, Sidney. *The Drug Dilemma*. New York: McGraw-Hill, 1969.

Cohen, Sidney. *Drugs of Hallucination*. London: Paladin, 1973.

Cook, Bruce. *The Beat Generation*. New York: Scribners, 1971.

Cookson, John, and Nottingham, Judith. *A Survey of Chemical and Biological Warfare.* New York: Monthly Review Press, 1969.

Corson, William R. *Armies of Ignorance: The Rise of the American Intelligence Empire.* New York: Dial Press, 1977.

DeRopp, Robert S. *Drugs and the Mind.* New York: Grove Press, 1961.

Dick, Philip. *The Three Stigmata of Palmer Eldritch.* New York: New American Library, 1964.

Dick, Philip. *A Scanner Darkly.* New York: New American Library, 1977.

Dickstein, Morris. *Gates of Eden: American Culture in the Sixties.* New York: Basic Books, 1977.

Didion, Joan. *Slouching Towards Bethlehem.* New York: Simon and Schuster, 1979.

Dormer, Frank J. *The Age of Surveillance: The Aims and Methods of America's Political Intelligence System.* New York: Vintage, 1981.

Dun, R. A. *Poetic Vision and the Psychedelic Experience.* Syracuse, New York: Syracuse University Press, 1970.

Ebin, David, ed. *The Drug Experience.* New York: Grove Press, 1965.

Eisen, Jonathan, ed. *The Age of Rock.* New York: Random House, 1969.

Epstein, Edward J. *Agency of Fear.* New York: Putnam, 1977.

Eszterhas, Joe. *Nark!* San Francisco: Straight Arrow Books, 1974.

Evans, Arthur. *Witchcraft and the Gay Counter-Culture.* Boston: Fag Rag Books, 1978.

Farina, Richard. *Been Down So Long It Looks Like Up to Me.* New York: Dell, 1971.

Felton, David, ed. Mindfuckers: *A Source Book on the Rise of Acid Fascism in America.* San Francisco: Straight Arrow Books, 1972.

216

Fort, Joel. *The Pleasure Seekers: The Drug Crisis, Youth and Society*. Indianapolis:Bobbs-Merrill, 1969.

Friedman, Myra. *Buried Alive: The Biography of Janis Joplin*. New York: Bantam, 1974.

Frith, Simon. *Sound Effects*. New York: Pantheon, 1981.

Fuller, John C. *The Day of St. Anthony's Fire*. New York: Macmillan, 1968.

Furst, Peter T. *Hallucinogens and Culture*. San Francisco: Chandler &. Sharp, 1976.

Gaskin, Stephen. *Amazing Dope Tales and Haight Street Flashbacks*. Summerton, Tennessee: The Book Publishing Company, 1980.

Geller, Allen, and Boas, Maxwell. *The Drug Beat*. New York: McGraw-Hill, 1969.

Gerzon, Mark. *The Whole World is Watching*. New York: Paperback Library, 1970.

Ginsberg, Allen. *Allen Verbatim*. New York: McGraw-Hill, 1975.

Ginsberg, Allen. *Composed on the Tongue*. Bolinas, California: Grey Fox Press, 1980.

Ginsberg, Allen. *Howl and Other Poems*. San Francisco: City Lights, 1956.

Ginsberg, Allen. *Kaddish and Other Poems 1958-60*. San Francisco: City Lights, 1961.

Ginsberg, Allen. *Planet News 1961-1967*. San Francisco: City Lights, 1968.

Ginsberg, Allen. Poems All Over the Place, Mostly 'Seventies. Cherry Valley Editions, 1978.

Gitlin, Todd. *The Whole World is Watching: Mass Media in the Making and Unmaking of the New Left*. Berkeley: University of California Press, 1980.

Gleason, Ralph. *The Jefferson Airplane and the San Francisco Sound*. New York: Ballantine, 1969.

Goldstein, Richard, *1 in 7; Drugs on Campus*. New York: Walker and Company, 1966.

Goldstein, Robert Justin. *Political Repression in Modern America*: 1870 to the Present. Cambridge, Massachusetts: Schenkman Publishing Co., 1978.

Goodman, Mitchell, ed. *The Movement Toward a New America*. New York: Pilgrim Press, 1970.

Greenfield, Robert. *The Spiritual Supermarket: An Account of Gurus Gone Public*. New York: Saturday Review Press, 1975.

Grinspoon, Lester, and Bakalar, James B. *Psychedelic Drugs Reconsidered*. New York: Basic Books, 1979.

Grof, Stanislov. *Realms of the Human Unconscious*. New York: Viking, 1975.

Grof, Stanislov, and Halifax, Joan. *The Human Encounter With Death*. New York: Dutton, 1978.

Grogan, Emmett. Ringolevio, *A Life Played for Keeps*. London: Heinemann, 1972.

Halperin, Morton H., et al. *The Lawless State: The Crimes of the U.S. Intelligence Agencies*. New York: Penguin, 1976.

Hamalian, Leo, and Karl, Frederick R., eds. *The Radical Vision*. New York: Thomas Y. Crowell Co., 1970.

Hamer, Michael J., ed. *Hallucinogens and Shamanism*. London: Oxford University Press, 1973. Hayes, Harold, ed. Smiling Through the Apocalypse. New York: Delta, 1971.

Hebidge, Dick. *Subculture: The Meaning of Style*. London: Methuen, 1979.

Henderson, David. *'Sense Me While I Kiss the Sky: The Life of Jimi Hendrix*. New York: Bantam, 1983.

Hersh, Burton. *The Mellon Family: A Fortune in History*. New York: William Morrow, 1978.

Hersh, *Seymour M. Chemical and Biological Warfare: America's Hidden Arsenal*. New York: Doubleday, 1969.

Hinckle, Warren. *If You Have a Lemon, Make Lemonade*. New York: Bantam, 1976.

Hofmann, Abbie. *Revolution for the Hell of It.* New York: Pocket Books, 1970.

Hofmann, Abbie. *Soon To Be a Major Motion Picture.* New York: Perigee, 1980.

Hofmann, Abbie. *Woodstock Nation.* New York: Vintage, 1969.

Hofmann, Abbie, and Hofmann, Anita. *To America with Love.* New York: Stonehill, 1976.

Hermann, Albert. *LSD: My Problem Child.* New York: McGraw-Hill, 1980.

Hollander, Charles, ed. *Student Drug Involvement.* Washington, DC: The National Student Association, 1967.

Hollingshead, Michael. *The Man Who Turned on the World.* London: Blond & Briggs, 1973.

Hopkins, Jerry, ed. *The Hippie Papers*, New York: Signet, 1968.

Herman, Richard E., and Fox, Allen M. *Drug Awareness: Key Documents on LSD, Marijuana, and the Drug Culture.* New York: Avon, 1970. Hougan, Jim. Decadence. New York: William Morrow, 1975.

Hougan, Jim. Spooks: The Haunting of America—The Private Use of Secret Agents. New York: William Morrow, 1978.

Howe, Irving. *Beyond the New Left.* New York: Horizon Press, 1965.

Huxley, Aldous. *Brave New World.* New York: The Modem Library, 1952.

Huxley, Aldous. *Brave New World Revisited.* New York: Bantam, 1960.

Huxley, Aldous. *Doors of Perception.* New York: Perennial Library, 1970.

Huxley, Aldous. *Heaven and Hell.* New York: Harper, 1956.

Huxley, Aldous. *Island.* New York: Bantam, 1971.

Huxley, Aldous. *Moksha: Writings on Psychedelics and the Visionary Experience (1931-1963).* Michael Horowitz and Cynthia Palmer, eds. New York: Stonehill, 1977.

Huxley, Aldous. *The Perennial Philosophy*. New York: Meridian Books, 1967.

Huxley, Laura Archera. *The Timeless Moment*. New York: Farrar, Straus and Giroux, 1968.

Hyde, Margaret O. *Mind Drugs*. New York: McGraw-Hill, 1973.

Inglis, Brian. *The Forbidden Game: A Social History of Drugs*. London: Hodder & Stoughton, 1975.

Jacobs, Harold, ed. *Weatherman*. Palo Alto: Ramparts Press, 1970.

Jacobs, Paul, and Landau, Saul. *The New Radicals: A Report with Documents*. New York: Vintage, 1966.

James, William. *The Varieties of Religious Experience*. New York: Modem Library, 1929.

Kerouac, Jack. *The Dharma Bums*. New York: Viking, 1958.

Kerouac, Jack. *On the Road*. New York: Viking, 1957.

Kesey, Ken. *One Flew Over the Cuckoo's Nest*. New York: Viking, 1962.

Kesey, Ken. *Ken Kesey's Garage Sale*. New York: Viking, 1973.

Kleps, Art. *The Boohoo Bible*. San Cristobal: The Toad Press, 1971.

Kleps, Art. *Millbrook*. Oakland: The Bench Press, 1975.

Kombluth, Jesse, ed. *Notes From the New Underground*. New York: Ace Publishing Corporation, 1968.

Koskoff, David E. *The Mellons: The Chronicle of America's Richest Family*. New York: Crowell, 1978.

Krassner, Paul, ed. *Best of the Realist*. Philadelphia: Running Press, 1984.

Krim, Seymour. *Shake It For the World*. Smartass, New York: Delta, 1971.

Kruger, Henrik. *The Great Heroin Coup: Drugs. Intelligence, & International Fascism*. Boston: South End Press, 1980.

Kuhn, Thomas. *The Structure of Scientific Revolutions*. Chicago: University of Chicago Press, 1970.

Laing, R.D. *The Politics of Experience and the Bird of Paradise.* London: Penguin, 1967.

Lamb, F. Bruce. *Wizard of the Upper Amazon.* Boston: Houghton Mifflin, 1974.

Lasby, Charles G. *Project Paperclip: German Scientists and the Cold War.* New York: Atheneum, 1971.

La Valley, Albert J., ed. *The New Consciousness.* Cambridge, Massachusetts: Winthrop Publishers, 1972.

Leary, Timothy. *Confessions of a Hope Fiend.* New York: Bantam, 1973.

Leary, Timothy. *Flashbacks: An Autobiography.* Los Angeles: J.P. Tarcher, 1983.

Leary, Timothy. *High Priest.* Cleveland: World Publishing Company, 1968.

Leary, Timothy, *Fall Notes.* New York: Douglas Book Corporation, 1970.

Leary, Timothy. *The Politics of Ecstasy.* London: Paladin, 1970.

Leary, Timothy. *Psychedelic Prayers.* Kerhonkson, New York: Poets Press, 1966.

Leary, Timothy. *What Does Woman Want?* Beverly Hills: 88 Books, 1976.

Leary, Timothy, Metzner, Ralph, and Alpert, Richard. *The Psychedelic Experience.* Secaucus: The Citadel Press, 1970.

Leary Timothy, with Wilson, Robert Anton, and Koopman, George A. *Neuropolitics.* Los Angeles: Starseed/Peace Press, 1977.

Lee, Dick, and Pratt, Colin. *Operation Julie.* London: W. H. Allen, 1978.

Legman, G. *The Fake Revolt.* New York: Breaking Point, 1967.

Lem, Stanislas. *The Futurological Congress.* New York: Seabury Press, 1974.

Lennard, Henry L. and associates. *Mystification and Drug Abuse.* New York: Harper &. Row, 1971.

Lerner, Michael P. *The New Socialist Revolution.* New York: Delacorte Press, 1973.

Lemoux, Penny. *In Banks We Trust.* New York: Anchor Press, 1984.

Lewis, Roger, *Outlaws of America.* London: Penguin, 1972.

Lilly, John. *The Scientist: A Novel Autobiography.* Philadelphia: Lippincott, 1978.

Lingeman, Richard R. *Drugs From A to Z: A Dictionary.* New York: McGraw-Hill, 1974.

London, Perry. *Behavior Control.* New York: New American Library, 1977.

Lothstein, Arthur, ed. *"All We Are Saying ..." The Philosophy of the New Left.* New York: Capricorn Books, 1970.

Louria, Donald. *Nightmare Drugs.* New York: Pocket Books, 1966.

Lukas, J. Anthony. *Don't Shoot—We Are Your Children!* New York: Random House, 1971.

Mailer, Norman. *The Armies of the Night.* New York: Signet, 1968.

Mailer, Norman. *Miami and the Siege of Chicago.* New York: Signet, 1968.

Mailer, Norman. *Pieces and Pontifications.* Boston: Little, Brown, 1982.

Mairowitz, David Zane. *The Radical Soap Opera: Roots of Failure in the American Left.* New York: Avon, 1976.

Marchetti, Victor, and Marks, John D. *The CIA and the Cult of Intelligence.* New York: Dell, 1974.

Marks, John. *The Search for the "Manchurian Candidate."* New York: Times Books, 1979.

Marsh, Dave, and Stein, Kevin. *The Book of Rock Lists.* New York: Dell, 1981.

Masters, R.E.L. and Houston, Jean. *The Varieties of Psychedelic Experience.* New York: Holt, Rinehart &. Winston, 1966.

McClure, Michael. *Meat Science Essays*. San Francisco: City Lights, 1970.

McCoy, Alfred W. *The Politics of Heroin in Southeast Asia*. New York: Harper Colophon Books, 1973.

McNeill, Don. *Moving Through Here*. New York: Lancer Books, 1970.

Meerloo, Joost A.M. *The Rape of the Mind*. New York: Grosset and Dunlap, 1961.

Melville, Keith. *Communes in the Counter Culture: Origins, Theories. Styles of Life*. New York: William Morrow, 1972.

Metzner, Ralph. *The Ecstatic Adventure*. New York: Macmillan, 1968.

Michaux, Henri. *The Major Ordeals of the Mind and the Countless Minor Ones*. New York: Harcourt Brace Jovanovich, 1974.

Michaux, Henri, *Miserable Miracle*. San Francisco: City Lights, 1963.

Miles. *Bob Dylan In His Own Words*. New York: Quick Fox, 1978.

Miller, Richard. *Bohemia: The Protoculture Then and Now*. Chicago: Nelson-Hall, 1977.

Mungo, Raymond. *Famous Long Ago: My Life and Hard Times with the Liberation News Service*. New York: Pocket Books, 1971.

Nahal, Chaman, ed. *Drugs and the Other Self: An Anthology of Spiritual Transformations*. New York: Harper &. Row, 1971.

Naranjo, Claudio. *The Healing Journey*. New York: Ballantine, 1975.

Newfield, Jack. *A Prophetic Minority*. New York: Signet Books, 1967.

Newland, Constance A. *My Self and I*. New York: Coward-McCann, 1962.

Norman, Philip. *Shout!* New York: Wamer Books, 1981.

Nowlis, Helen H. *Drugs on the College Campus*. New York: Anchor Books, 1969.

Nuttall, Jeff. *Bomb Culture*. London: Paladin, 1970.

Oglesby, Carl, and Shaull, Richard. *Containment and Change*. New York: Macmillan, 1967.

Oglesby, Carl, ed. *The New Left Reader*. New York: Grove Press, 1969.

Olson, Charles. *I Maximus* (Volume I). Bolinas, California: Four Seasons Foundation, 1977.

O'Neill, William L. *Coming Apart*. Chicago: Quadrangle, 1971.

Papworth, M.H. *Human Guinea Pigs*. Boston: Beacon Press, 1967.

Paz, Octavio. *Alternating Current*. New York: Viking, 1973.

Perkus, Cathy. *COINTELPRO: The FBI's Secret War on Political Freedom*. New York: Monad Press, 1975.

Perry, Charles. *The Haight-Ashbury: A History*. New York: Random House, 1984.

Pichaske, David. *A Generation in Motion: Popular Music and Culture in the Sixties*. New York: Schirmer Books, 1979.

Picon, Gaeton. *Surrealists and Surrealism*. New York: Rizzoli, 1983.

Poirier, Richard. *The Performing Self: Compositions and Decompositions in the Languages of Contemporary Life*. New York: Oxford University Press, 1971.

Pope, Harrison, Jr. *Voices from the Drug Culture*. Boston: Beacon Press, 1974.

Portuges, Paul. The Visionary Poetics of Allen Ginsberg. Santa Barbara: Ross-Erikson, 1978.

Powers, Thomas. *The Man Who Kept the Secrets*. New York: Pocket Books, 1981.

Pynchon, Thomas. *Gravity's Rainbow*. New York: Viking, 1973.

Raskin, Jonah. *Out of the Whale: Growing Up in the American*

Left. New York: Links Books, 1974.

Reich, Charles. *The Greening of America*. New York: Random House, 1970.

Rips, Geoffrey. *Unamerican Activities: The Campaign Against the Underground*, Press. San Francisco: City Lights, 1981.

The editors of Rolling Stone. *The Age of Paranoia*. New York: Pocket Books, 1972.

Roseman, Bernard. *LSD; The Age of the Mind*. Hollywood: Wilshire Book Company, 1963.

Rossman, Michael. *New Age Blues: On the Politics of Consciousness*. New York: E.P. Dutton, 1979.

Rossman, Michael. *On Learning and Social Change*. New York: Vintage, 1972.

Rossman, Michael. *Wedding Within the War*. New York: Doubleday, 1971.

Roszak, Theodore. *The Making of a Counter Culture*. New York: Anchor Books, 1969.

Rubin, Jerry. *Do It!* New York: Simon and Schuster, 1970.

Rubin, Jerry. *Growing (Up) at 37*. New York: Wamer Books, 1976.

Rubin, Jerry. *We Are Everywhere*. New York: Harper Colophon Books, 1971.

Ruether, Rosemary. *The Radical Kingdom*. New York: Paulist Press, 1970.

Sale, Kirkpatrick. *SDS*. New York: Vintage, 1974.

Sanders, Ed. *The Family*. New York: Dutton, 1972.

Sanders, Ed. *Shards of God*. New York: Grove Press, 1970.

Sayres, Sohnya, Stephanson, Anders, Aronowitz, Stanley, and Jameson, Fredric, eds. *The 60s Without Apology*. Minneapolis: University of Minnesota Press, 1984.

Scaduto, Anthony. *Dylan*. New York: Grosset and Dunlap, 1971.

Scheflin, Alan W, and Opton, Edward M., Jr. *The Mind Manipulators*. New York: Paddington Press, 1978.

Schein, Edgar. *Coercive Persuasion*. New York: W. W. Norton, 1971.

Schrag, Peter. *Mind Control*. New York: Pantheon, 1978.

Sheed, Wilfred. *Clare Boothe Luce*. New York: Dutton, 1982.

Siegel, Ronald K., and West, L. J., eds. *Hallucinations: Behavior, Experience, and Theory*. New York: John Wiley, 1975.

Sinclair, John. *Guitar Army*. New York: Douglas Book Corporation, 1972. Situationist International. Point Blank! Berkeley, 1972.

Slack, Charles W. *Timothy Leary, the Madness of the Sixties*, and Me. New York: Peter H. Wyden, 1974.

Sloman, Larry. Reefer Madness. New York: Bobbs-Merrill, 1979.

Smith, David, ed. *The New Social Drug*. Englewood Cliffs, New Jersey: Prentice-Hall, 1970.

Smith, David E., and Luce, John. *Love Needs Care*. Boston: Little Brown, 1971.

Smith, Huston. *Forgotten Truth: The Primordial Tradition*. New York: Harper & Row, 1976.

Smith, R. Harris. *OSS; The Secret History of America's First Central Intelligence Agency*. New York: Delta, 1973.

Solomon, David, ed. *LSD: The Consciousness-Expanding Drug*. New York: Berkeley-Medallion, 1966.

Solomon, David, ed. *The Marijuana Papers*. New York: Mentor, 1968.

Spellman, A.B. *Four Lives in the Be-Bop Business*. New York: Pantheon, 1966.

Spitz, Robert Stephen. *Barefoot in Babylon*. New York: Viking, 1979.

Stafford, P.G. and Golightly, B.H. *LSD: The Problem-Solving Psychedelic*. New York: Award Books, 1967.

Stafford, Peter. *Psychedelic Baby Reaches Puberty*. New York: Delta, 1971.

Stafford, Peter. *Psychedelics Encyclopedia*. Los Angeles: J.P. Tarcher, 1983.

Stensill, Peter, and Mairowitz, David Zane, eds. BAMN (By Any Means Necessary): *Outlaw Manifestos and Ephemera 1965-70*. London: Penguin, 1971. Stone, Robert. Dog Soldiers. Boston: Houghton Mifflin, 1973.

Swanberg, W.A. *Luce and His Empire*. New York: Charles Scribner's Sons, 197.

Szasz, Thomas. *Ceremonial Chemistry*. New York: Anchor Press, 1975.

Tart, Charles T. *On Being Stoned*. Palo Alto: Science and Behavior Books, 1971.

Taussig, Michael. *The Devil and Commodity Fetishism in South America*. Chapel Hill: University of North Carolina Press, 1983.

Taylor, Norman. *Flight From Reality*. New York: Duell, Sloane and Pearce, 1949.

Tendler, Stewart, and May, David. *The Brotherhood of Eternal Love*. London: Panther Books, 1984.

Teodori, Massimo, ed. *The New Left: A Documentary History*. Indianapolis: Bobbs-Merrill, 1969.

Thomas, J.C. *Chasin' the Trane*. New York: Doubleday, 1975.

Thompson, Hunter S. *Fear and Loathing in Las Vegas*. New York: Popular Library, 1971.

Thompson, Hunter S. *The Great Shark Hunt*. New York: Summit Books, 1979.

Thompson, Hunter S. *Hell's Angels*. New York: Ballantine, 1966.

Viorst, Milton. *Fire in the Streets: America in the 1960s*. New York: Simon and Schuster, 1979.

von Hofmann, Nicholas. *We Are the People Our Parents Warned Us Against*. Greenwich, Connecticut: Fawcett Publications, 1973.

Wakefield, Dan. *The Addict*. Greenwich, Connecticut: Fawcett Publications, 1963.

Wasson, R. Gordon, Ruck, Carl A.R, and Hofmann, Albert. *The*

Road to Eleusis:

Unveiling the Secrets of the Mysteries. New York: Harcourt Brace Jovanovich, 1978.

Wasson, R. Gordon. *Soma: Divine Mushroom of Immortality.* New York: Harcourt, Brace &. World, 1968.

Watts, Alan W. *The Joyous Cosmology*. New York: Pantheon, 1962.

Well, Andrew. *The Natural Mind*. Boston: Houghton Mifflin, 1972.

Well, Gunther M., Metzner, Ralph, and Leary, Timothy, eds. *The Psychedelic Reader.*

Secaucus, New Jersey: The Citadel Press, 1973.

Weiner, Rex, and Stillman, Deanne. *Woodstock Census*. New York: Viking, 1979.

Wells, Brian. *Psychedelic Drugs*. Baltimore: Penguin, 1973.

Wiener, John. *Come Together: John Lennon in His Time*. New York: Random House, 1984.

Wilkinson, Paul. *The New Fascists*. London: Pan Books, 1983.

Wolf, Leonard. *Voices from the Love Generation*. Boston: Little, Brown, 1968.

Wolfe, Burton H. *The Hippies*. New York: New American Library, 1968.

Wolfe, Tom. *The Electric Kool-Aid Acid Test*. New York: Bantam, 1969.

Yablonsky, Lewis. *The Hippie Trip*. Baltimore: Penguin, 1973.

Young, Warren, and Hixson, Joseph. *LSD on Campus*. New York: Dell, 1966.

Zaroulis, Nancy, and Sullivan, Gerald. *Who Spoke Up?,* New York: Doubleday, 1984.

U.S. Government Reports—

Alleged Assassination Plots Involving Foreign Leaders. An Interim Report of the Select Committee to Study Governmental Operations with respect to IntelligenceActivities, United States Senate, November 20, 1975.

Biomedical and Behavioral Research, 1975. Joint Hearings before the Subcommittee on Health of the Committee on Labor and Public Welfare and the Subcommittee on Administrative Practice and Procedure of the Committee on the Judiciary, United States Senate, September 10, 12; and November 7, 1975.

Chemical, Biological and Radiological Warfare Agents. Hearings before the Committee on Science and Astronautics. United States House of Representatives, June 16 and 22, 1959.

C1A: The Pike Report. Nottingham: Spokesman Books, 1977.

The C1A and the Media. Hearings before the Subcommittee on Oversight of the Permanent Select Committee on Intelligence, House of Representatives, December 27, 28, and 29, 1977; January 4, 5; and April 20, 1978.

Drug Safety. Hearings before a Subcommittee of the Committee on Government Operations, House of Representatives, March 9, 10; May 25, 26; June 7, 8 and 9, 1966.

Final Report of the Select Committee to Study Governmental Operations with Respect to Intelligence Activities. United States Senate, Books I-VI.

Hashish Smuggling and Passport Fraud: The Brotherhood of Eternal Love. Hearings before the Subcommittee to Investigate the Administration of the Internal Security Act and other Internal Security Laws of the Senate Judiciary Committee, 1973.

Human Drug Testing by the C1A, 1977. Hearings before the Subcommittee on Health and Scientific Research of the Committee on Human Resources, United States Senate.

Individual Rights and the Federal Role in Behavior Modification. A Study Prepared by the Staff of the Subcommittee on Constitutional Rights by the Committee on the Judiciary, United States Senate, 1974.

The Narcotic Rehabilitation Act of 1966. Hearings before a Special Subcommittee of the Committee on the Judiciary, United States Senate, January 25-27; May 12, 13, 19, 23 and 25; June 14-15; July 19 1966.

The Nelson Rockefeller Report to the President. Commission on CIA Activities. New York: Manor Books, 1975.

Organization and Coordination of Federal Drug Research and Regulatory Programs: LSD. Hearings before the Subcommittee on Executive Reorganization of the Committee on Government Operations, United States Senate, May 24-26, 1966.

Project MK-ULTRA, The CIA's Program of Research in Behavior Modification. Joint Hearing before the Select Committee on Intelligence and the Subcommittee on Health and Scientific Research of the Committee on Human Resources, United States Senate, August 3, 1977.

Unauthorized Storage of Toxic Agents. Hearings before the Select Committee to Study Governmental Operations with respect to Intelligence Activities of the United States Senate, Volume 1, September 16-18, 1975.

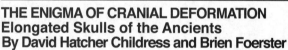

Get these fascinating books from your nearest bookstore or directly from:
Adventures Unlimited Press
www.adventuresunlimitedpress.com

COVERT WARS AND BREAKAWAY CIVILIZATIONS
By Joseph P. Farrell

Farrell delves into the creation of breakaway civilizations by the Nazis in South America and other parts of the world. He discusses the advanced technology that they took with them at the end of the war and the psychological war that they waged for decades on America and NATO. He investigates the secret space programs currently sponsored by the breakaway civilizations and the current militaries in control of planet Earth. Plenty of astounding accounts, documents and speculation on the incredible alternative history of hidden conflicts and secret space programs that began when World War II officially "ended."
292 Pages. 6x9 Paperback. Illustrated. $19.95. Code: BCCW

THE ENIGMA OF CRANIAL DEFORMATION
Elongated Skulls of the Ancients
By David Hatcher Childress and Brien Foerster

In a book filled with over a hundred astonishing photos and a color photo section, Childress and Foerster take us to Peru, Bolivia, Egypt, Malta, China, Mexico and other places in search of strange elongated skulls and other cranial deformation. The puzzle of why diverse ancient people—even on remote Pacific Islands—would use head-binding to create elongated heads is mystifying. Where did they even get this idea? Did some people naturally look this way—with long narrow heads? Were they some alien race? Were they an elite race that roamed the entire planet? Why do anthropologists rarely talk about cranial deformation and know so little about it? Color Section.
250 Pages. 6x9 Paperback. Illustrated. $19.95. Code: ECD

ARK OF GOD
The Incredible Power of the Ark of the Covenant
By David Hatcher Childress

Childress takes us on an incredible journey in search of the truth about (and science behind) the fantastic biblical artifact known as the Ark of the Covenant. This object made by Moses at Mount Sinai—part wooden-metal box and part golden statue—had the power to create "lightning" to kill people, and also to fly and lead people through the wilderness. The Ark of the Covenant suddenly disappears from the Bible record and what happened to it is not mentioned. Was it hidden in the underground passages of King Solomon's temple and later discovered by the Knights Templar? Was it taken through Egypt to Ethiopia as many Coptic Christians believe? Childress looks into hidden history, astonishing ancient technology, and a 3,000-year-old mystery that continues to fascinate millions of people today. Color section.
420 Pages. 6x9 Paperback. Illustrated. $22.00 Code: AOG

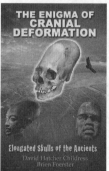

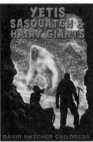

YETIS, SASQUATCH & HAIRY GIANTS
By David Hatcher Childress
Childress takes the reader on a fantastic journey across the Himalayas to Europe and North America in his quest for Yeti, Sasquatch and Hairy Giants. Childress begins with a discussion of giants and then tells of his own decades-long quest for the Yeti in Nepal, Sikkim, Bhutan and other areas of the Himalayas, and then proceeds to his research into Bigfoot, Sasquatch and Skunk Apes in North America. Chapters include: The Giants of Yore; Giants Among Us; Wildmen and Hairy Giants; The Call of the Yeti; Kanchenjunga Demons; The Yeti of Tibet, Mongolia & Russia; Bigfoot & the Grassman; Sasquatch Rules the Forest; Modern Sasquatch Accounts; more. Includes a 16-page color photo insert of astonishing photos!
360 pages. 5x9 Paperback. Illustrated. Bibliography. Index. $18.95. Code: YSHG

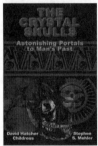

SECRETS OF THE HOLY LANCE
The Spear of Destiny in History & Legend
by Jerry E. Smith
Secrets of the Holy Lance traces the Spear from its possession by Constantine, Rome's first Christian Caesar, to Charlemagne's claim that with it he ruled the Holy Roman Empire by Divine Right, and on through two thousand years of kings and emperors, until it came within Hitler's grasp—and beyond! Did it rest for a while in Antarctic ice? Is it now hidden in Europe, awaiting the next person to claim its awesome power? Neither debunking nor worshiping, *Secrets of the Holy Lance* seeks to pierce the veil of myth and mystery around the Spear.
312 PAGES. 6x9 PAPERBACK. ILLUSTRATED. $16.95. CODE: SOHL

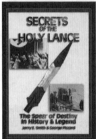

THE CRYSTAL SKULLS
Astonishing Portals to Man's Past
by David Hatcher Childress and Stephen S. Mehler
Childress introduces the technology and lore of crystals, and then plunges into the turbulent times of the Mexican Revolution form the backdrop for the rollicking adventures of Ambrose Bierce, the renowned journalist who went missing in the jungles in 1913, and F.A. Mitchell-Hedges, the notorious adventurer who emerged from the jungles with the most famous of the crystal skulls. Mehler shares his extensive knowledge of and experience with crystal skulls. Having been involved in the field since the 1980s, he has personally examined many of the most influential skulls, and has worked with the leaders in crystal skull research. Color section.
294 pages. 6x9 Paperback. Illustrated. $18.95. Code: CRSK

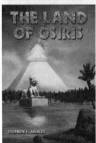

THE LAND OF OSIRIS
An Introduction to Khemitology
by Stephen S. Mehler
Was there an advanced prehistoric civilization in ancient Egypt? Were they the people who built the great pyramids and carved the Great Sphinx? Did the pyramids serve as energy devices and not as tombs for kings? Chapters include: Egyptology and Its Paradigms; Khemitology—New Paradigms; Asgat Nefer—The Harmony of Water; Khemit and the Myth of Atlantis; The Extraterrestrial Question; more. Color section.
272 PAGES. 6x9 PAPERBACK. ILLUSTRATED . $18.95. CODE: LOOS

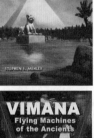

VIMANA:
Flying Machines of the Ancients
by David Hatcher Childress
According to early Sanskrit texts the ancients had several types of airships called vimanas. Like aircraft of today, vimanas were used to fly through the air from city to city; to conduct aerial surveys of uncharted lands; and as delivery vehicles for awesome weapons. David Hatcher Childress, popular *Lost Cities* author, takes us on an astounding investigation into tales of ancient flying machines. In his new book, packed with photos and diagrams, he consults ancient texts and modern stories and presents astonishing evidence that aircraft, similar to the ones we use today, were used thousands of years ago in India, Sumeria, China and other countries. Includes a 24-page color section.
408 Pages. 6x9 Paperback. Illustrated. $22.95. Code: VMA

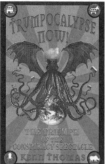

TRUMPOCALYPSE NOW!
The Triumph of the Conspiracy Spectacle
by Kenn Thomas

Trumpocalypse Now! takes a look at Trump's career as a conspiracy theory celebrity, his trafficking in such notions as birtherism, Islamofascism and 9/11, the conspiracies of the Clinton era, and the JFK assassination. It also examines the controversies of the 2016 election, including the cyber-hacking of the DNC, the Russian involvement and voter fraud. Learn the parapolitcal realities behind the partisan divide and the real ideological underpinnings behind the country's most controversial president. Chapters include: Introduction: Alternative Facts; Conspiracy Celebrity–Trump's TV Career; Birtherism; 9/11 and Islamofascism; Clinton Conspiracies; JFK–Pro-Castro Fakery; Cyber Hacking the DNC; The Russian Connection; Votescam; Conclusion: Alternative Theories; more.

6x9 Paperback. 380 Pages. Illustrated. $16.95. Code: TRPN

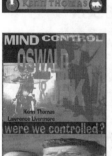

MIND CONTROL, OSWALD & JFK
Introduction by Kenn Thomas

In 1969 the strange book *Were We Controlled?* was published which maintained that Lee Harvey Oswald was a special agent who was also a Mind Control subject who had received an implant in 1960. Thomas examines the evidence that Oswald had been an early recipient of the Mind Control implant technology and this startling role in the JFK Assassination. Also: the RHIC-EDOM Mind Control aspects concerning the RFK assassination and the history of implant technology.

256 Pages. 6x9 Paperback. Illustrated. $16.00. Code: MCOJ

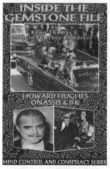

INSIDE THE GEMSTONE FILE
Howard Hughes, Onassis & JFK
By Kenn Thomas & David Childress

Here is the low-down on the most famous underground document ever circulated. Photocopied and distributed for over 20 years, the Gemstone File is the story of Bruce Roberts, the inventor of the synthetic ruby widely used in laser technology today, and his relationship with the Howard Hughes Company and ultimately with Aristotle Onassis, the Mafia, and the CIA. Hughes kidnapped and held a drugged-up prisoner for 10 years; Onassis and his role in the Kennedy Assassination; how the Mafia ran corporate America in the 1960s; more.

320 Pages. 6x9 Paperback. Illustrated. $16.00. Code: IGF

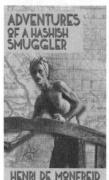

ADVENTURES OF A HASHISH SMUGGLER
by Henri de Monfreid

Nobleman, writer, adventurer and inspiration for the swashbuckling gun runner in the *Adventures of Tintin*, Henri de Monfreid lived by his own account "a rich, restless, magnificent life" as one of the great travelers of his or any age. The son of a French artist who knew Paul Gaugin as a child, de Monfreid sought his fortune by becoming a collector and merchant of the fabled Persian Gulf pearls. He was then drawn into the shadowy world of arms trading, slavery, smuggling and drugs. Infamous as well as famous, his name is inextricably linked to the Red Sea and the raffish ports between Suez and Aden in the early years of the twentieth century. De Monfreid (1879 to 1974) had a long life of many adventures around the Horn of Africa where he dodged pirates as well as the authorities.

284 Pages. 6x9 Paperback. $16.95. Illustrated. Code AHS

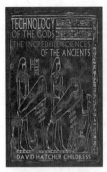

TECHNOLOGY OF THE GODS
The Incredible Sciences of the Ancients
by David Hatcher Childress

Childress looks at the technology that was allegedly used in Atlantis and the theory that the Great Pyramid of Egypt was originally a gigantic power station. He examines tales of ancient flight and the technology that it involved; how the ancients used electricity; megalithic building techniques; the use of crystal lenses and the fire from the gods; evidence of various high tech weapons in the past, including atomic weapons; ancient metallurgy and heavy machinery; the role of modern inventors such as Nikola Tesla in bringing ancient technology back into modern use; impossible artifacts; and more.

356 pages. 6x9 Paperback. Illustrated. $16.95. code: TGOD

THE ANTI-GRAVITY HANDBOOK
edited by David Hatcher Childress

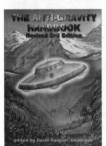

The new expanded compilation of material on Anti-Gravity, Free Energy, Flying Saucer Propulsion, UFOs, Suppressed Technology, NASA Cover-ups and more. Highly illustrated with patents, technical illustrations and photos. This revised and expanded edition has more material, including photos of Area 51, Nevada, the government's secret testing facility. This classic on weird science is back in a new format!

230 PAGES. 7X10 PAPERBACK. ILLUSTRATED. $16.95. CODE: AGH

ANTI–GRAVITY & THE WORLD GRID

Is the earth surrounded by an intricate electromagnetic grid network offering free energy? This compilation of material on ley lines and world power points contains chapters on the geography, mathematics, and light harmonics of the earth grid. Learn the purpose of ley lines and ancient megalithic structures located on the grid. Discover how the grid made the Philadelphia Experiment possible. Explore the Coral Castle and many other mysteries, including acoustic levitation, Tesla Shields and scalar wave weaponry. Browse through the section on anti-gravity patents, and research resources.

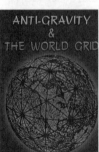

274 PAGES. 7X10 PAPERBACK. ILLUSTRATED. $14.95. CODE: AGW

ANTI–GRAVITY & THE UNIFIED FIELD
edited by David Hatcher Childress

Is Einstein's Unified Field Theory the answer to all of our energy problems? Explored in this compilation of material is how gravity, electricity and magnetism manifest from a unified field around us. Why artificial gravity is possible; secrets of UFO propulsion; free energy; Nikola Tesla and anti-gravity airships of the 20s and 30s; flying saucers as superconducting whirls of plasma; anti-mass generators; vortex propulsion; suppressed technology; government cover-ups; gravitational pulse drive; spacecraft & more.

240 PAGES. 7X10 PAPERBACK. ILLUSTRATED. $14.95. CODE: AGU

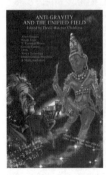

THE TIME TRAVEL HANDBOOK
A Manual of Practical Teleportation & Time Travel
edited by David Hatcher Childress

The Time Travel Handbook takes the reader beyond the government experiments and deep into the uncharted territory of early time travellers such as Nikola Tesla and Guglielmo Marconi and their alleged time travel experiments, as well as the Wilson Brothers of EMI and their connection to the Philadelphia Experiment—the U.S. Navy's forays into invisibility, time travel, and teleportation. Childress looks into the claims of time travelling individuals, and investigates the unusual claim that the pyramids on Mars were built in the future and sent back in time. A highly visual, large format book, with patents, photos and schematics. Be the first on your block to build your own time travel device!

316 PAGES. 7X10 PAPERBACK. ILLUSTRATED. $16.95. CODE: TTH

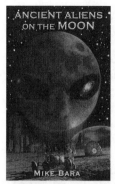

ANCIENT ALIENS ON THE MOON
By Mike Bara
What did NASA find in their explorations of the solar system that they may have kept from the general public? How ancient really are these ruins on the Moon? Using official NASA and Russian photos of the Moon, Bara looks at vast cityscapes and domes in the Sinus Medii region as well as glass domes in the Crisium region. Bara also takes a detailed look at the mission of Apollo 17 and the case that this was a salvage mission, primarily concerned with investigating an opening into a massive hexagonal ruin near the landing site. Chapters include: The History of Lunar Anomalies; The Early 20th Century; Sinus Medii; To the Moon Alice!; Mare Crisium; Yes, Virginia, We Really Went to the Moon; Apollo 17; more. Tons of photos of the Moon examined for possible structures and other anomalies.
248 Pages. 6x9 Paperback. Illustrated.. $19.95. Code: AAOM

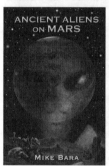

ANCIENT ALIENS ON MARS
By Mike Bara
Bara brings us this lavishly illustrated volume on alien structures on Mars. Was there once a vast, technologically advanced civilization on Mars, and did it leave evidence of its existence behind for humans to find eons later? Did these advanced extraterrestrial visitors vanish in a solar system wide cataclysm of their own making, only to make their way to Earth and start anew? Was Mars once as lush and green as the Earth, and teeming with life? Chapters include: War of the Worlds; The Mars Tidal Model; The Death of Mars; Cydonia and the Face on Mars; The Monuments of Mars; The Search for Life on Mars; The True Colors of Mars and The Pathfinder Sphinx; more. Color section.
252 Pages. 6x9 Paperback. Illustrated. $19.95. Code: AMAR

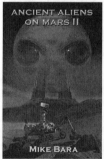

ANCIENT ALIENS ON MARS II
By Mike Bara
Using data acquired from sophisticated new scientific instruments like the Mars Odyssey THEMIS infrared imager, Bara shows that the region of Cydonia overlays a vast underground city full of enormous structures and devices that may still be operating. He peels back the layers of mystery to show images of tunnel systems, temples and ruins, and exposes the sophisticated NASA conspiracy designed to hide them. Bara also tackles the enigma of Mars' hollowed out moon Phobos, and exposes evidence that it is artificial. Long-held myths about Mars, including claims that it is protected by a sophisticated UFO defense system, are examined. Data from the Mars rovers Spirit, Opportunity and Curiosity are examined; everything from fossilized plants to mechanical debris is exposed in images taken directly from NASA's own archives.
294 Pages. 6x9 Paperback. Illustrated. $19.95. Code: AAM2

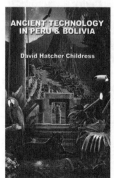

ANCIENT TECHNOLOGY IN PERU & BOLIVIA
By David Hatcher Childress
Childress speculates on the existence of a sunken city in Lake Titicaca and reveals new evidence that the Sumerians may have arrived in South America 4,000 years ago. He demonstrates that the use of "keystone cuts" with metal clamps poured into them to secure megalithic construction was an advanced technology used all over the world, from the Andes to Egypt, Greece and Southeast Asia. He maintains that only power tools could have made the intricate articulation and drill holes found in extremely hard granite and basalt blocks in Bolivia and Peru, and that the megalith builders had to have had advanced methods for moving and stacking gigantic blocks of stone, some weighing over 100 tons.
340 Pages. 6x9 Paperback. Illustrated.. $19.95 Code: ATP

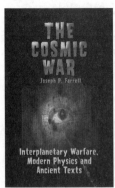
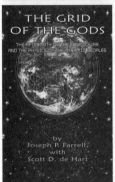
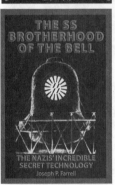
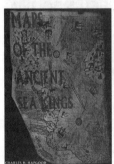

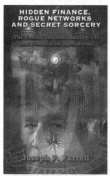

HIDDEN FINANCE, ROGUE NETWORKS & SECRET SORCERY
The Fascist International, 9/11, & Penetrated Operations
By Joseph P. Farrell

Pursuing his investigations of high financial fraud, international banking, hidden systems of finance, black budgets and breakaway civilizations, Farrell investigates the theory that there were not *two* levels to the 9/11 event, but *three*. He says that the twin towers were downed by the force of an exotic energy weapon, one similar to the Tesla energy weapon suggested by Dr. Judy Wood, and ties together the tangled web of missing money, secret technology and involvement of portions of the Saudi royal family. Farrell unravels the many layers behind the 9-11 attack, layers that include the Deutschebank, the Bush family, the German industrialist Carl Duisberg, Saudi Arabian princes and the energy weapons developed by Tesla before WWII.
296 Pages. 6x9 Paperback. Illustrated. $19.95. Code: HFRN

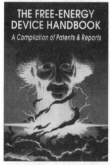

THRICE GREAT HERMETICA AND THE JANUS AGE
By Joseph P. Farrell

What do the Fourth Crusade, the exploration of the New World, secret excavations of the Holy Land, and the pontificate of Innocent the Third all have in common? Answer: Venice and the Templars. What do they have in common with Jesus, Gottfried Leibniz, Sir Isaac Newton, Rene Descartes, and the Earl of Oxford? Answer: Egypt and a body of doctrine known as Hermeticism. The hidden role of Venice and Hermeticism reached far and wide, into the plays of Shakespeare (a.k.a. Edward DeVere, Earl of Oxford), into the quest of the three great mathematicians of the Early Enlightenment for a lost form of analysis, and back into the end of the classical era, to little known Egyptian influences at work during the time of Jesus.
354 Pages. 6x9 Paperback. Illustrated. $19.95. Code: TGHJ

THE FREE-ENERGY DEVICE HANDBOOK
A Compilation of Patents and Reports
by David Hatcher Childress

A large-format compilation of various patents, papers, descriptions and diagrams concerning free-energy devices and systems. *The Free-Energy Device Handbook* is a visual tool for experimenters and researchers into magnetic motors and other "over-unity" devices. With chapters on the Adams Motor, the Hans Coler Generator, cold fusion, superconductors, "N" machines, space-energy generators, Nikola Tesla, T. Townsend Brown, and the latest in free-energy devices. Packed with photos, technical diagrams, patents and fascinating information, this book belongs on every science shelf.
292 PAGES. 8x10 PAPERBACK. ILLUSTRATED. $16.95. CODE: FEH

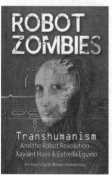

ROBOT ZOMBIES
Transhumanism and the Robot Revolution
By Xaviant Haze and Estrella Eguino,

Technology is growing exponentially and the moment when it merges with the human mind, called "The Singularity," is visible in our imminent future. Science and technology are pushing forward, transforming life as we know it—perhaps even giving humans a shot at immortality. Who will benefit from this? This book examines the history and future of robotics, artificial intelligence, zombies and a Transhumanist utopia/dystopia integrating man with machine. Chapters include: Love, Sex and Compassion—Android Style; Humans Aren't Working Like They Used To; Skynet Rises; Blueprints for Transhumans; Kurzweil's Quest; Nanotech Dreams; Zombies Among Us; Cyborgs (Cylons) in Space; Awakening the Human; more. Color Section.
180 Pages. 6x9 Paperback. Illustrated. $16.95. Code: RBTZ

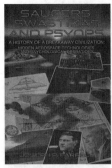

SAUCERS, SWASTIKAS AND PSYOPS
A History of a Breakaway Civilization
By Joseph P. Farrell
Farrell discusses SS Commando Otto Skorzeny; George Adamski; the alleged Hannebu and Vril craft of the Third Reich; The Strange Case of Dr. Hermann Oberth; Nazis in the US and their connections to "UFO contactees"; The Memes—an idea or behavior spread from person to person within a culture—are Implants. Chapters include: The Nov. 20, 1952 Contact: The Memes are Implants; The Interplanetary Federation of Brotherhood; Adamski's Technological Descriptions and Another ET Message: The Danger of Weaponized Gravity; Adamski's Retro-Looking Saucers, and the Nazi Saucer Myth; Dr. Oberth's 1968 Statements on UFOs and Extraterrestrials; more.
272 Pages. 6x9 Paperback. Illustrated. $19.95. Code: SSPY

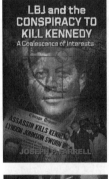

LBJ AND THE CONSPIRACY TO KILL KENNEDY
By Joseph P. Farrell
Farrell says that a coalescence of interests in the military industrial complex, the CIA, and Lyndon Baines Johnson's powerful and corrupt political machine in Texas led to the events culminating in the assassination of JFK. Chapters include: Oswald, the FBI, and the CIA: Hoover's Concern of a Second Oswald; Oswald and the Anti-Castro Cubans; The Mafia; Hoover, Johnson, and the Mob; The FBI, the Secret Service, Hoover, and Johnson; The CIA and "Murder Incorporated"; Ruby's Bizarre Behavior; The French Connection and Permindex; Big Oil; The Dead Witnesses: Guy Bannister, Jr., Mary Pinchot Meyer, Rose Cheramie, Dorothy Killgallen, Congressman Hale Boggs; LBJ and the Planning of the Texas Trip; LBJ: A Study in Character, Connections, and Cabals; LBJ and the Aftermath: Accessory After the Fact; The Requirements of Coups D'État; more.
342 Pages. 6x9 Paperback. $19.95 Code: LCKK

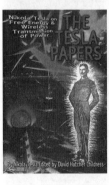

THE TESLA PAPERS
Nikola Tesla on Free Energy &
Wireless Transmission of Power
by Nikola Tesla, edited by David Hatcher Childress
David Hatcher Childress takes us into the incredible world of Nikola Tesla and his amazing inventions. Tesla's fantastic vision of the future, including wireless power, anti-gravity, free energy and highly advanced solar power. Also included are some of the papers, patents and material collected on Tesla at the Colorado Springs Tesla Symposiums, including papers on: •The Secret History of Wireless Transmission •Tesla and the Magnifying Transmitter •Design and Construction of a Half-Wave Tesla Coil •Electrostatics: A Key to Free Energy •Progress in Zero-Point Energy Research •Electromagnetic Energy from Antennas to Atoms
325 PAGES. 8x10 PAPERBACK. ILLUSTRATED. $16.95. CODE: TTP

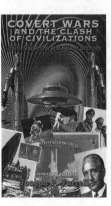

COVERT WARS & THE CLASH OF CIVILIZATIONS
UFOs, Oligarchs and Space Secrecy
By Joseph P. Farrell
Farrell's customary meticulous research and sharp analysis blow the lid off of a worldwide web of nefarious financial and technological control that very few people even suspect exists. He elaborates on the advanced technology that they took with them at the "end" of World War II and shows how the breakaway civilizations have created a huge system of hidden finance with the involvement of various banks and financial institutions around the world. He investigates the current space secrecy that involves UFOs, suppressed technologies and the hidden oligarchs who control planet earth for their own gain and profit.
358 Pages. 6x9 Paperback. Illustrated. $19.95. Code: CWCC

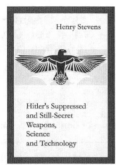

HITLER'S SUPPRESSED AND STILL-SECRET WEAPONS, SCIENCE AND TECHNOLOGY
by Henry Stevens

In the closing months of WWII the Allies assembled mind-blowing intelligence reports of supermetals, electric guns, and ray weapons able to stop the engines of Allied aircraft—in addition to feared x-ray and laser weaponry. Chapters include: The Kammler Group; German Flying Disc Update; The Electromagnetic Vampire; Liquid Air; Synthetic Blood; German Free Energy Research; German Atomic Tests; The Fuel-Air Bomb; Supermetals; Red Mercury; Means to Stop Engines; more.
335 Pages. 6x9 Paperback. Illustrated. $19.95. Code: HSSW

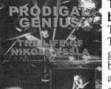

PRODIGAL GENIUS
The Life of Nikola Tesla
by John J. O'Neill

This special edition of O'Neill's book has many rare photographs of Tesla and his most advanced inventions. Tesla's eccentric personality gives his life story a strange romantic quality. He made his first million before he was forty, yet gave up his royalties in a gesture of friendship, and died almost in poverty. Tesla could see an invention in 3-D, from every angle, within his mind, before it was built; how he refused to accept the Nobel Prize; his friendships with Mark Twain, George Westinghouse and competition with Thomas Edison. Tesla is revealed as a figure of genius whose influence on the world reaches into the far future. Deluxe, illustrated edition.
408 pages. 6x9 Paperback. Illustrated. Bibliography.
$18.95. Code: PRG

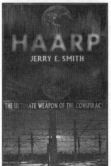

HAARP
The Ultimate Weapon of the Conspiracy
by Jerry Smith

The HAARP project in Alaska is one of the most controversial projects ever undertaken by the U.S. Government. At at worst, HAARP could be the most dangerous device ever created, a futuristic technology that is everything from super-beam weapon to world-wide mind control device. Topics include Over-the-Horizon Radar and HAARP, Mind Control, ELF and HAARP, The Telsa Connection, The Russian Woodpecker, GWEN & HAARP, Earth Penetrating Tomography, Weather Modification, Secret Science of the Conspiracy, more. Includes the complete 1987 Eastlund patent for his pulsed super-weapon that he claims was stolen by the HAARP Project.
256 pages. 6x9 Paperback. Illustrated. Bib. $14.95. Code: HARP

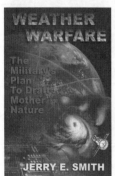

WEATHER WARFARE
The Military's Plan to Draft Mother Nature
by Jerry E. Smith

Weather modification in the form of cloud seeding to increase snow packs in the Sierras or suppress hail over Kansas is now an everyday affair. Underground nuclear tests in Nevada have set off earthquakes. A Russian company has been offering to sell typhoons (hurricanes) on demand since the 1990s. Scientists have been searching for ways to move hurricanes for over fifty years. In the same amount of time we went from the Wright Brothers to Neil Armstrong. Hundreds of environmental and weather modifying technologies have been patented in the United States alone – and hundreds more are being developed in civilian, academic, military and quasi-military laboratories around the world *at this moment!* Numerous ongoing military programs do inject aerosols at high altitude for communications and surveillance operations.
304 Pages. 6x9 Paperback. Illustrated. Bib. $18.95. Code: WWAR

ORDER FORM

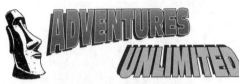

One Adventure Place
P.O. Box 74
Kempton, Illinois 60946
United States of America
Tel.: 815-253-6390 • Fax: 815-253-6300
Email: auphq@frontiernet.net
http://www.adventuresunlimitedpress.com

ORDERING INSTRUCTIONS

✓ Remit by USD$ Check, Money Order or Credit Card

✓ Visa, Master Card, Discover & AmEx Accepted

✓ Paypal Payments Can Be Made To:

    info@wexclub.com

✓ Prices May Change Without Notice

✓ 10% Discount for 3 or More Items

SHIPPING CHARGES

United States

✓ Postal Book Rate { $4.50 First Item / 50¢ Each Additional Item

✓ POSTAL BOOK RATE Cannot Be Tracked!
Not responsible for non-delivery.

✓ Priority Mail { $6.00 First Item / $2.00 Each Additional Item

✓ UPS { $7.00 First Item / $1.50 Each Additional Item

NOTE: UPS Delivery Available to Mainland USA Only

Canada

✓ Postal Air Mail { $15.00 First Item / $2.50 Each Additional Item

✓ Personal Checks or Bank Drafts MUST BE
US$ and Drawn on a US Bank

✓ Canadian Postal Money Orders OK

✓ Payment MUST BE US$

All Other Countries

✓ Sorry, No Surface Delivery!

✓ Postal Air Mail { $19.00 First Item / $6.00 Each Additional Item

✓ Checks and Money Orders MUST BE US$
and Drawn on a US Bank or branch.

✓ Paypal Payments Can Be Made in US$ To:
info@wexclub.com

SPECIAL NOTES

✓ RETAILERS: Standard Discounts Available

✓ BACKORDERS: We Backorder all Out-of-
Stock Items Unless Otherwise Requested

✓ PRO FORMA INVOICES: Available on Request

✓ DVD Return Policy: Replace defective DVDs only

ORDER ONLINE AT: www.adventuresunlimitedpress.com

**10% Discount When You Order
3 or More Items!**

Please check: ✓

☐ This is my first order   ☐ I have ordered before

Name

Address

City

State/Province   Postal Code

Country

Phone: Day   Evening

Fax   Email

Item Code	Item Description	Qty	Total

Please check: ✓

☐ Postal-Surface

☐ Postal-Air Mail
(Priority in USA)

☐ UPS
(Mainland USA only)

☐ Visa/MasterCard/Discover/American Express

Subtotal ▶	
Less Discount-10% for 3 or more items ▶	
Balance ▶	
Illinois Residents 6.25% Sales Tax ▶	
Previous Credit ▶	
Shipping ▶	
Total (check/MO in USD$ only) ▶	

Card Number:

Expiration Date: Security Code:

✓ SEND A CATALOG TO A FRIEND: